GW01071876

RACHEL
MY GALLANT SOLDIER

RACHEL
MY GALLANT SOLDIER

SUSAN DAVIES

A Deirdre McDonald Book
London

First published in 1995 by
Deirdre McDonald Books
128 Lower Richmond Road
London SW15 1LN

Designed by Mick Keates

ISBN 1 898094 04 7

Phototypeset by Intype, London

**Printed and bound in Great Britain by
Hartnolls Limited, Bodmin, Cornwall**

DEDICATIONS

To Rachel:
she fought so hard.

To Peter (my backbone):
without your love and support I would never have coped.

To Katy:
thank you for being you. You'll never know how much
you helped me, allowing me to support Rachel to the
full, sometimes to the detriment of your own needs,
with no word of complaint.

To our parents:
you were always there, especially when we needed you most.

Thank you one and all. I love you.

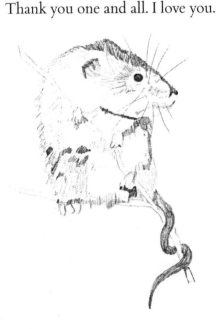

Foreword

This is a story of a very brave little girl, written
with love and devotion by her mother.
Rachel's story is filled with courage, tears and
laughter. She had a ready smile for anyone
who came her way. The story was written in
the hope that others faced with a similar
situation would be able to gain some
understanding of the techniques used and the
choices that have to be made in the
treatment of cancer.
Rachel touched our lives so briefly but
brought great joy. She lost her fight
but left a legacy of memories. Her courage
was an inspiration to all who knew her.

Katharine

H.R.H. The Duchess of Kent

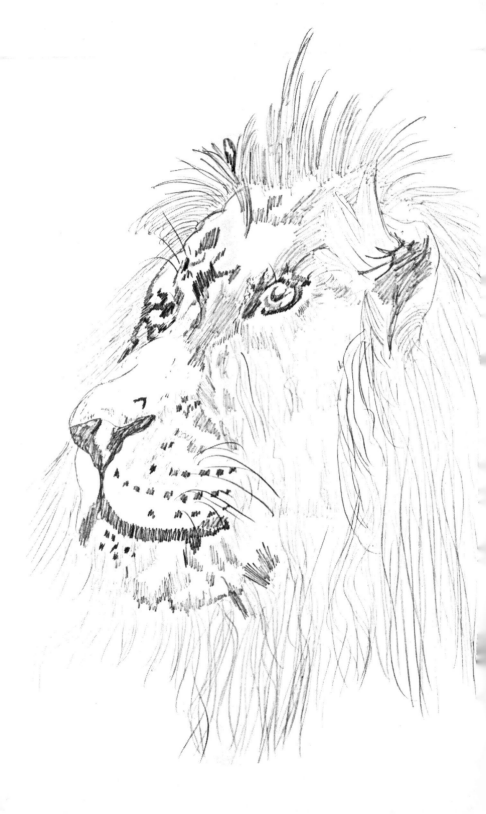

PREFACE

WHEN SOMEONE YOU LOVE is diagnosed with a terminal illness, your world just folds, you are in a state of panic, your mind is in a turmoil; but at the same time you need to be calm. There are so many questions you need answers to and you suddenly find yourself in the mysterious world of medicine.

Within the following pages you will learn of the courage of a special young lady – my daughter Rachel. You will read of how she coped with traumatic treatments, how a very ordinary family was turned upside down, and of how our love for each other pulled us through.

The treatment of cancer is a very complex procedure and while the medical profession does its best to explain the various techniques, there comes a time when you simply have to trust and have faith in your team of doctors, praying that they have the magic formula that will work.

All I can do now is to relay to you, from a mother's point of view, my daughter's experiences and hope that you will find it helpful should you be experiencing the same or similar in your life.

CHAPTER ONE

RACHEL CAME INTO the world at 8.50 on the morning of 2 April 1975, weighing a healthy 8lb 3oz. The midwife propped me up to see her being born. After checking her all over and being content that she was all right (because every woman has a secret fear that her baby will not be quite perfect), I thought my worries were over. She was perfect in every way. Now I could enjoy this new little treasure along with my other little treasure, her sister Katy, nearly two years her senior, and bring them up through a happy and loving childhood until they became adults and went out into the big wide world to live their own lives.

The years went rolling by. They learned to walk and talk and did all the usual things that babies and toddlers do. Then they started school. Soon they had to cope with an experience that not every child has to face. When Rachel was five and Katy was seven, their father John and I separated. This was in January 1981, and we divorced soon afterwards. When I remarried in August 1982 the girls accepted Peter, my new husband, very well and he them, and life started to be wonderful again. We bought a new home and they started new schools, settling in easily, quickly making new friends, and our house was soon full of children playing and having tea. We had holidays abroad and many carefree, happy days when we did just as we pleased – until January 1985.

For nine years Rachel had been a normal, healthy, happy little girl, having only the usual childhood diseases. Always on the plump side, but very agile, she enjoyed all the things children love – swimming, rollerbooting, walking, bike-riding, horse-riding – and was never still for a minute. She was also a very loving child, always thinking of others, always ready to help someone less fortunate than herself.

In November 1984 Rachel first complained of a pain in her left leg. She had just returned from a birthday party which was, in her words, 'brill', and was demonstrating a new skill she had acquired – break-dancing – so I immediately put the aching leg down to a strain and told her that after a good night's rest and paracetomol all would be well. But next morning she woke up still in pain and our usually cheerful little girl was most unhappy and constantly crying. For Rachel to be miserable was so out of character that Pete and I decided to take her to the local hospital casualty department (it was a weekend). The doctor who examined her said he thought she had an infected hair follicle and prescribed a course of penicillin. He said that if it did not improve in a few days we should take her to our GP. After a few days the ache seemed to go away and Rachel returned to her usual self, battling about the house like a sherman tank, so life returned to normal.

December came with all the usual hustle and bustle and the excitement of school concerts and parties. We had a lovely Christmas with all the family. January started with snowmen and sledging and then back to school for another term of hard work. Rachel loved school and was extremely bright for her age, her favourite subject being music. She played the recorder and obtained grades for her playing from the Trinity School of Music in London. Our house was never quiet, because at that time Katy was also a keen musician, and

4

both girls liked to practise different pieces at the same time, trying to outdo each other in the way that brothers and sisters always do. Pete and I would eventually have to call for silence.

January 26 was a Saturday. Rachel woke up with leg ache again. This time I went to the local health centre, thinking that she had another infection. Our usual doctor was not there, and the locum on duty seemed offhand, suggesting that there was nothing wrong with Rachel and that she was merely seeking attention. I tried to explain that this had happened to her before and that a course of antibiotics seemed to make it better, but he was adamant that there was nothing wrong and refused to listen to me. I was furious that he had suggested Rachel was putting it on. He did not know my child; I did.

I took Rachel home again, and all I could give her for her pain was paracetomol, but this was just a temporary measure. On Monday we went back to the health centre and saw our own GP who could see at a glance there was something very wrong with Rachel simply because she was so unhappy. Because he could not see or feel anything untoward, he recommended an X-ray at the Kent and Sussex Hospital and sent us there immediately. At this stage, although I was worried by Rachel's pain, I felt confident that it must be something relatively simple, such as a green-stick fracture.

At the hospital casualty department the doctors listened to what had gone before and confirmed that an X-ray would be a good idea. Rachel was frightened at the prospect because she had only ever been in hospital to visit others, but they explained to her all about X-rays and she agreed to go ahead. The picture showed an abnormality in Rachel's left tibia (shin bone). They couldn't be sure what it was, but one

5

suggestion was that it might be osteomylitis (an infection in the bone). Blood tests were taken and then the doctor came to see me and said that Rachel would have to be admitted. My stomach turned a somersault and I began to feel frightened.

Rachel had never been away from us before, except to visit her Gran or Aunty Ann or Daddy, and the thought of having to stay in a strange place on her own naturally frightened her. I was told I could stay with her until she settled in, so I rang home and asked Pete to bring some things to the hospital. 'Tell Dad not to forget Mumice,' Rachel said (Mumice was a very special toy rabbit that she had had since she was six months old), 'I can't sleep without him.' Peter doesn't drive so he had to recruit a friend to bring him to the hospital. The friend's wife looked after Katy while he was gone.

At first we were told that she would be in for a few days while tests were carried out. These 'few days' turned into four weeks, during which Rachel underwent many different tests. A bone scan was arranged at Pembury Hospital. They grew cultures with her blood, which took about ten days, and then the scan had to be reported on. Still we were none the wiser. The doctors then decided that a biopsy should be taken from the bone. We had to explain to Rachel that she was going to have an operation. She was not at all impressed with this and said she was frightened and wanted to go home. I felt the same way, but we were assured by the doctors that it was a minor operation, purely routine, and then they would have some definite results for us. Feeling very frustrated and helpless, we went ahead. We just wanted her better and back home with us again.

All went well with the operation. Rachel was very good and made no fuss, except when she came back from theatre because, of course, she was sore. She became very noisy during her recovery from the anaesthetic and all her inhibitions seemed to go. The nurses told us it happens quite often. On reflection she was quite funny, but at the time I was very distressed to see her so upset. The next day she was back to normal, sporting a plaster cast on her leg, which she thought was 'brill'. She had settled quite well into the hospital routine, revelling in the constant stream of visitors and presents. On constant bed-rest, she became her normal cheerful self, regaling her visitors with all the gory details of the operation.

I can't remember the exact date when I was told Rachel had cancer, but I know it was a Friday. Pete had asked me if I wanted him to come with me to the hospital to see the doctors, but I was so confident that they weren't going to tell me anything terrible that I sent him off to work saying, 'If you don't hear from me by 3 P.M., everything is all right.' I took Katy to school then went on to the hospital to stay with Rach, as I did every day until other visitors and family came to give me a break.

Rachel's father, John, and I had an appointment with the consultant at lunchtime. When he came into the room, we were told to sit down, and he said he did not have good news for us. Rachel had Ewings Sarcoma, a bone cancer, and we would have to go to London for the latest treatment. I can remember thinking, what does he think he's saying? He's got the wrong patient's notes. Old people have cancer, not children. The consultant said he couldn't explain much about the treatment as it was not in his field, we would have to put any questions to the doctors in London. At the time I felt numb, but my head was spinning. I remember someone giving me a cup of tea. I remember crying, and then I remember thinking: 'What can I tell Rachel? What will

Pete say? How am I going to tell my Mum and Dad, her grandparents, and what about Katy. What can I say to Aunty Ann and Uncle Rod? On and on went the questions, until I realized that I had to go back to the ward and play with Rachel as if everything was all right; I couldn't fall apart now. I dried my eyes, washed my face and reapplied my make-up. I made the decision not to telephone Peter as I knew that as soon as I heard his voice I would crumple, and for now I had to be strong. John said goodbye to Rachel, saying he would see her later, and Rachel and I played normally until my Mum and Dad came to visit so I could be at home when Katy returned from school.

I don't remember driving home to Paddock Wood (about a fifteen-minute drive), but when I put my key in the front door I doubled up, and cried and cried. Katy came home from school and asked me what was wrong, but I couldn't explain it to her; I just told her that Rachel was going to be in hospital for a good while longer and the thought of it had upset me. I sent her off to do some shopping. Meanwhile 3 P.M. had come and gone with no word from me, so Peter in London assumed everything was all right. When he arrived home he found me distraught. We talked it over and spoke to our parents and, still in a state of shock, went back to the hospital to see Rachel and tuck her up for the night.

We were allowed to take Rachel home for the weekend before she was to be transferred to the Westminster Hospital in London. We had a lovely weekend. It was nice just to be together again after nearly a month. Peter and I discussed Rachel's illness at length and decided that she must be told both what was wrong with her, and as much as we knew, which wasn't a lot, about the treatment. We explained to Rachel that she had a bone tumour and that she would have to have a drug treatment known as chemotherapy; it would

8

make her feel ill but at the same time it would make her better. She cried and said she was frightened, but realized that if she wanted to get better it was something she would have to go through. We told her that she could die from the tumour if it was left untreated. She said, 'I've got to have it done, I don't want to die.'

It was an impossible situation, one you can never be ready for. Who would expect to have to discuss such things with their child? We were all crying and feeling trapped, but in her usual manner Rachel said, 'Come on, don't let's cry any more. Let's forget about it.' We got on with our nice weekend together.

We returned to the Kent and Sussex for our transfer to the Westminster Hospital by ambulance, saying goodbye to all the nurses and other patients and the many friends Rachel had made of the domestic staff and porters. She was already quite famous as she had appeared on TVS news, with another child called Simon, in a feature about some old tiles that had been found on the walls of her ward during refurbishing work. We were able to video it and she loved to show everyone when they came to visit.

CHAPTER TWO

WE WERE ADMITTED to Princess Margaret Rose Ward in the Westminster Hospital on 27 February 1985 and introduced to our Consultant Mr Hanam and the Senior Registrar Dr Andy Stockdale. Andy and Rachel were to become great friends. He was very forthright with us all. We told him that we had explained everything we could to Rachel about her illness, but that we had not used the word cancer. He said he understood and proceeded to tell us in great detail about chemotherapy and its side-effects. He told Rachel she would lose her hair; he told her he was going to make her very sick, and that by the end of the treatment, which was going to last for nearly twelve months, she would hate the sight of him, but he felt confident he could take her pain away and hoped to make her better.

We were also offered a mid-thigh amputation followed by chemotherapy. We were told to talk it through with each other and then with Rachel. This we did and decided we would like to try the chemotherapy and radiotherapy, as we felt that an amputation was so final, and even then they could not guarantee an absolute cure; Rachel could develop a secondary elsewhere.

We discussed all of this with a little girl of nine years old and asked her what she felt about it. It was hard enough for us to understand and cope with, and yet we knew we couldn't put her through all that lay ahead without knowing how she felt about things. Neither of the choices seemed very inviting, but when the alternative is death, they begin to look quite good. Rachel was adamant that she did not want to have her leg amputated so we made the decision to go ahead with the regime of chemotherapy and radiotherapy.

It was all systems go from the time we were admitted to the Westminster. The tests were carried out swiftly and all the information possible was given to us to help us feel a little bit more in control. During this time Rachel settled down to making friends and the best of a not-very-nice situation as only she could; she had the nurses and doctors in fits of laughter with her antics.

By 4 March Rachel was ready for her first dose of chemotherapy, having undergone another operation on 1 March to have a Hickman Line inserted into her chest. This is a catheter inserted into a main artery which enables the doctors to administer drugs and take blood samples without having constantly to be sticking needles into their patients, causing even more distress. Although at first I was apprehensive about my daughter having a strange tube fixed into her, I soon realized it was a wonderful invention. Gone was the little girl who gritted her teeth and trembled when it was time for a blood test; it was lovely to see her happy and smiling, chatting and making jokes. A treatment such as chemotherapy requires so many blood tests to check levels of red and white cells that this seemed to be the ideal solution to cut down distress and bruising. The Hickman had to be flushed through twice a day with an anti-coagulant drug called hepsal which kept the line free from blood-clotting, giving the doctors a clear channel for their treatments. When caring for the Hickman, stringent hygiene had to be observed – rubber gloves, masks and so on were worn – as it can very easily become a source of infection.

The next step was the first administering of the highly toxic drugs into our little girl. Knowing the side-effects was bad enough, but at this stage no one could tell how Rachel was going to react to the drugs. All sorts of mixed thoughts went racing through my mind. The doctor entered the room holding a tray containing eight or nine syringes filled with various coloured liquids. My stomach lurched. The doctor looked so young, a boy almost. Did he really know what he was doing? How could someone so young be allowed to do such complicated and dangerous procedures to my baby? What if he makes a mistake? My mind was a whirl of uncertainty. I wanted to take Rachel away from all this. I wanted to say stop, I've changed my mind!

The doctor explained to us what the drugs in the syringes were called and what they were supposed to do. He told Rachel that he had a sleeping drug called lorazepam which he would administer to her through her Hickman Line. When she was fast asleep he would then give her all the other drugs and when she woke up it would all be over – except that she would probably feel sick. Rachel was a bit tearful, which was understandable, but her attitude was 'Just get on with it, put me to sleep and let's get it over with'.

The doctor began. He injected the lorazepam very slowly, watching Rachel carefully. Gradually she began to relax and drifted off to sleep. She began to twitch and, when I asked why, he explained that her body was relaxing and that there was nothing to worry about. After Rachel was fully asleep he proceeded to empty the syringes into her one after the other. The whole process took about half an hour. I can remember feeling so frightened and unsure, and praying that we were doing the right thing. The doctor knew how I was feeling and tried to reassure me all the time, but I was battling with an almost uncontrollable urge to push him away and say 'No more!' Peter was aware of this and held on to me tightly. He told me to trust the doctor, that Rachel had faith in what was being done and that I must have that same faith. Of course he was right, and I was so pleased he was there with me, but I don't think I have ever been so scared as I was that night.

After Rachel had been given her drugs she continued to sleep peacefully. Peter went home to Paddock Wood and our other daughter Katy, who was being looked after at home by mum and dad. I went back to Rachel and slept next to her bed in case she woke in the night. The nurses came in and out all through the night to monitor her. Next morning Rachel woke and said she felt sick. She was sick and then went back to sleep. This continued all that day; at times the retching was so violent that her little face turned purple and the veins on her face and neck stood out. The nurses gave her injections of an anti-sickness drug called Maxolon which calmed it down a lot but didn't stop it completely.

By the evening Rachel was keeping awake for longer periods in between the vomiting attacks, and said she was feeling a little better. She began to take sips of water. She was kept on a saline drip so that she didn't dehydrate. She was so relieved that it was all over. I was so proud of her and told her she was a very brave girl. The doctor came back to give her more drugs but this batch, he said, would not make her sick. She slept peacefully again all night, absolutely worn out from her vomiting day. The next morning she woke up feeling sore in her tummy from all the retching, but after a small breakfast she was soon bouncing around on her bed asking for sweets and a game of this and that. I was amazed and relieved to see the way she had coped and that she seemed so much better already.

After this first treatment the doctors were able to assess Rachel's tolerance to the chemotherapy. They also were very pleased with the results, and told us that we could go home at the end of the week minus the leg plaster. Rachel would have crutches so that the leg didn't have too much strain put on it; it would be weak for a while until the bone had a chance to replenish itself. Rachel was over the moon with this news, and couldn't wait to get home and see all the family and her friends.

We were told that the treatment Rachel had just undergone would have to be repeated every twenty-one days. Our routine was to be two days' hospitalization for the chemotherapy; seven days later a visit to the outpatients clinic for a check-up and a shot of a drug that would cause no side-effects, home again; seven days later, another visit to the clinic for a check-up and another shot of the same drug and home again; seven days later, two days' hospitalization for chemo – and so on. As we progressed through the regime we would have odd weeks when no outpatient treatment would be needed, so all in all it wasn't too bad. At least in between treatments and clinic visits we would all be at home together and Rachel could live a reasonably normal life. From the first dose of chemotherapy Rachel's pain subsided and she was back to her old mischievous self. It felt so good to have her back to being Rachel again.

With the news of Rachel being allowed home came the realization that her Hickman Line would still need to be flushed through twice a day. When I asked the doctors how this would be done – a district nurse perhaps? – I was told that I would do it, of course. My blood ran cold. How could I possibly do such a thing? I wasn't a nurse, and the thought of injecting Rachel's line at home on my own scared me to death. What if I made a mistake? The doctors told me that the ward sister would teach me how to do it while Rachel was still in hospital. I was to flush the line with the sister watching me until I had gained confidence. The first time I did it my hands wouldn't stop shaking, but the sister talked me through it and congratulated me when I had finished saying, 'Once you get the hang of it, it will be like brushing your teeth.' Fat chance of that, I thought, but she was right, although the first time I did it at home I was just as scared as the first time in the hospital. There was no sister there to talk me through it and Rachel was laughing at me and waving the end of the Hickman at me so that I couldn't get the syringe in. She trusted me completely, bless her. After I gained confidence I then taught Peter how to do it so that if any time I had a cold or wanted to go out he could do it for me.

Rachel's bedroom was like a mini-hospital ward with all the supplies they sent home with us: needles, syringes, gloves, masks and so on. Once when I was flushing Rachel's line she suddenly went limp, as if she had fainted. My heart missed a beat, then just as suddenly she burst out laughing and said, 'Don't panic, I'm only messing about.' The little monkey was always up to her tricks, but soon this procedure became a way of life and we didn't think twice about it.

So, newly proficient in the art of flushing Hickman Lines, and armed with a bag full of equipment, we were told we could go home. Rachel had been given instructions on how to use the crutches by the physiotherapist. She was still insisting that her leg was strong enough to walk on without crutches, but the doctors insisted and she was a good girl and accepted that she had to use them for a while. In fact, she was on crutches for about four months. They were a nuisance to her and gave her hands blisters but she was so intent on getting better she adapted her play-time games with no trouble and coped admirably in her usual way. Rachel never moaned about the things she couldn't do, but just made the best of what she could do and had a whale of a time. Her friends were great too and did not mind slowing things down a bit or helping her when she needed it.

One day we went for a check-up and Andy, the registrar, saw the way Rachel was using the crutches. 'For what little use they are to you, young lady, you might as well leave them here with me,' he said. She was so thrilled that she gave Andy a kiss, and said, 'See, I told you I didn't need them!' Andy's face showed he was just as thrilled to be able to give back to Rachel a little bit of her freedom.

As the treatment progressed Rachel was scanned regularly and an improvement could be seen, but at the same time she was building up resistance to the sleeping drug. Rachel took longer to be sedated, and became more aware of what was happening to her during the administration of the drugs. Each time she could remember a little more, and each time, understandably she became more apprehensive.

In all, Rachel had to undergo this treatment fifteen times, the first being 4 March 1985 and the last being 19 February 1986. Towards the end it proved very difficult indeed to get her to go. We made a countdown chart so that she could cross off the treatments as she completed them. We used to call them tumour-bashing days and make a joke about how scared the tumour must be every time she went into the hospital, knowing that it was slowly being destroyed. We were also guilty of bribing her with special treats of visits to places she wanted to see. This gave her something to look forward to, to spur her on to get into the hospital, get it

16

over with and get out as soon as possible to go wherever it was she had chosen.

During this time she also lost her hair. Even though you have had it explained to you and you know it is going to happen, when it actually does it is heart-breaking. It began to fall little by little, then in huge chunks. Finally one morning she came into our bedroom and said, 'Mum, can you brush my hair? It's all in a tangle.' It was a matted mess at the back of her head where she had lain on it in the night and as I began to untangle it the whole lot just came away in my hand. All four of us sat on our bed crying, but after the initial shock Rachel said it felt much better. She had had a beautiful head of hair and now it had all gone.

Rachel's hair loss was only going to be temporary, the doctors assured us. They said the new hair, when it grew, would probably be even better than before. They were right – her second head of hair came through exactly the same colour but the texture was unbelievable; it was also slightly wavy. Rachel was thrilled when it started to grow again, but for now she had no hair at all. In a special sort of way she looked lovely. The hospital provided her with a wig, a perfect match in colour and style. They worked very hard to make sure she had the best they had to offer and it was so good that few people were aware that she even wore one. She told her close friends and of course the family knew. After the initial shock of losing her hair Rachel even made jokes about wearing a wig. She called it the cat and frequently asked for a saucer of milk for it. She also used to do impressions with it and had us in hysterics with some of them, rolling the wig into a long sausage shape and putting it down the centre of her head pretending she was B.A. from 'The A-Team'. She thought it was great that she could have her hair washed by me in the bathroom while she watched television in the lounge. This irritated poor Katy who would have to miss television while I washed *her* hair.

Rachel used to make Granddad Davies laugh when he was visiting. She would suddenly disappear behind the settee and Granddad would say, 'What you doing, Rach?' and a little voice would say, 'I'm having a scratch.' Off would come the wig and scratching noises and little sighs of pleasure could be heard coming from behind the settee. The wig irritated her scalp sometimes when she got hot, but instead of letting it get her down she just sorted herself out in her usual down-to-earth manner.

It took a long time for Granddad Denton to be able to cope with Rachel's hair loss, it upset him so much. He couldn't bear to see what was happening to his granddaughter and often used to say, 'Why couldn't it have been me?' When he saw how well Rachel was coping and how she was always joking, he began to relax more. They had always been good buddies – Rachel had inherited her sense of fun from my Dad – and they were always teasing and playing tricks on one another. It was a relief to see him able to overcome his worries and treat her just as he had before her illness.

On windy days Rachel was always worried that the wig might blow away, so she used to wear a hat. Once when she was playing out in the street with one of her friends and her sister, a boy came up and said, 'Watcha, Rach, like yer hat,' and promptly grabbed it. Off came the wig too. At first Rachel began to cry and Katy was ready to protect her sister against any nasty jibes, but when the child saw what had happened he turned white. He was so afraid that he had pulled all Rachel's hair out that he had no thought of ridiculing her, and instead of Rachel needing comforting, the little boy had to be reassured that he had done her no harm. When they had explained it all to him he was very sympathetic and never once teased her or told anyone else, and they remained the best of friends. Kate and Rachel came indoors to tell us, thinking it was a terrific joke, and of course it did nothing but good for Rachel, giving her the confidence she needed. Her attitude to her illness was much the same as to the hair loss – she would make a joke about it. In hospital she would sometimes walk about with a sick bowl on her head as a hat (they were made of cardboard), and when the nurses said 'What are you doing with that on your head?' she would reply, 'It's there in case of an emergency.' She was a terrific child.

After several months of chemotherapy we had one or two hiccups with infections and problems with the Hickman. Chemotherapy knocks the immune system pretty hard and Rachel's white cell count would drop, leaving her wide open to infection. At these times we had to keep her away from people if they were unwell. She had a Hickman Line infection which laid her low for nearly a week and she was hospitalized on very high doses of penicillin. Once she had a urine infection which meant hospital for a week and very high doses of penicillin again, so we had to be very careful and monitor her quite closely.

On another occasion Rachel and Katy decided they would have a game of something which resulted in the usual sisterly disagreements, pushing and shoving. Accidentally Katy caught her hand in Rachel's Hickman Line. Trying to free herself she tugged it. Rachel screamed for help. Pete and I rushed in to find Katy on the point of collapse (she's very squeamish) and Rachel screaming, with blood running down her side. On investigation it was not as bad as it first appeared. The skin around the point of entry had torn slightly – hence the bleeding. After calming everyone down, peace reigned.

As you can see, our lives revolved around hospitals and

appointments and we were under considerable stress one way and another. But we had a good family behind us to help us constantly. When our three-weekly chemo trips began, my Mum and Dad would move into our home and look after Katy. I was able to forget about running the house and go to stay with Rachel. Peter, of course, had to keep his job going. In the following pages you will see how we spent our two days every three weeks.

CHAPTER THREE

RACHEL AND I would set off on a Wednesday morning, having said goodbye to Katy. Katy was such a good girl throughout; she never complained at being left, and I think my parents spoiled her a bit to make up for her not seeing us. I used to ring her in the evening to chat about her day.

When Rachel and I arrived at the hospital we would have the usual check-ups, see the doctors and consultant, pick up the chemotherapy drugs and then go to the Westminster Children's Hospital further along the road for the doctors there to administer the drugs. By now the Princess Margaret Rose Ward at the main Westminster Hospital had been closed down (it was the only children's ward in the hospital) and neither we nor the doctors felt it was right to treat a little girl on an adult cancer ward. Arrangements were therefore made for us to have the check-ups at the main hospital and the treatment at the children's hospital.

We would be admitted, usually late in the afternoon, on to Gomer Berry Ward. By this stage Rachel would be terrified and usually vomited when she walked on the ward. The nurses always greeted us with such friendliness that it was like a second home. We got to know them, the doctors, and many of the patients, because most of them were like Rachel and had a serious illness which needed constant treatment.

Rachel's father John would come to see her on Wednesday

evening, while Peter and I had supper. After John had gone home, Peter would stay with us until quite late. He always stayed with me while they gave Rachel her drugs because although we got a little more used to it as time passed, it was still a very daunting feeling watching such things happening to her. After the drugs were given Pete would go home to Paddock Wood, usually too late to see Katy. Invariably she would have left him a note asking for help with her homework. This he would do and leave her a note for the morning – poor Katy had a strange home life for a while.

After saying goodbye to Peter I would make up a bed in Rachel's cubicle and settle down for the night. Rachel usually slept until about 4 or 5 A.M., then she would wake temporarily, vomit and go back to sleep. That's how she would be all Thursday. The vomiting at the beginning of the treatment was relatively easy (if there is an easy way to be sick) but as the day progressed she used to retch so hard it was agony to watch.

Peter's Mum always came to see Rachel mid-afternoon on Thursday. By this time the sleeping drug would be starting to wear off and the sickness would be subsiding. This became a challenge for Rachel as she loved her Gran's visits. She would say to me: 'Gran will be here soon, I must get cleaned up.' They always made plans for what they were going to do – read or play a particular game – from one visit to the next so, weak as she was sometimes, she would have a wash, put on a clean nightie and be ready for Gran.

Some times were better than others. I have known her vomit for eighteen hours, at ten-minute intervals for the first five to six hours, then gradually the intervals would lengthen. Another time it would last for about seven hours. The doctors couldn't explain this, although they thought it might be something to do with Rachel's mental approach at that particular time. They said that they had noticed the same reactions in other patients too.

After Gran's visit, Pete would come straight from work and have a chat and game with Rachel. In the evening John would come so that Pete and I could go for some supper. That way Rachel was never left alone. After our supper, John would leave and then we waited for the next dose of drugs to be given. These would not upset Rachel because she knew they would not affect her like the previous night's drugs. Then she would settle down for a good night's sleep. Pete would go home and then I would settle down next to Rach for the night.

In the morning (Friday) Rachel would be like a rag doll, her tummy sore after the constant vomiting, but she would be determined that she was going home as soon as possible. She would have a cup of tea and, if that stayed down, she would nibble a piece of toast or have some cornflakes, then she would say, 'Come on, Mum, let's get out of here.' We would pack our things, say our goodbyes and thank yous and walk to Victoria Station. Rachel was still very fragile, but she liked to walk to the station as it was the first fresh air – if you can call London air fresh – for two days. Our first port of call was Casey Jones (a burger bar) on Victoria station and then we boarded the train for home with Rachel clutching her burger and milk-shake. By the time we reached Paddock Wood our little girl would bounce off the train to meet her Granddad who was waiting for us with open arms and the car. At home Gran would be waiting with a cup of tea and a bacon sandwich – Rachel's favourite snack, always requested before she left home on Wednesday. Off with her coat, on with the telly; Rachel would sit on her bean bag, bacon sandwich on her knee, cup of tea in her hand and be as happy as Larry. After a short rest she would rush all over

23

the place, catching up with things she had missed in the previous two days. That was the pattern of Rachel's two days in every three weeks.

When Katy came home from school, Gran and Granddad would say their goodbyes and the girls would go out in the street to play with their friends. Pete would come home from work (invariably he was greeted by Rachel and Katy outside) and it never ceased to amaze us how quickly Rachel dismissed hospitals and her treatment and fell straight back into her normal routine. We would stand at the window and watch her playing, and we would say to each other, 'Did the last two days really happen?' Peter and I would be exhausted, me from lack of sleep, and him from his constant travelling, and Rachel would be charging about as if nothing had happened. She used to make us feel quite ashamed sometimes – she seemed to cope so much better than we did.

Friday nights were Guide nights and Rachel would go to her meeting at 6.30 P.M., be home at 8, and then she would say, 'I think I'll go to bed now and have an early night because I've got to do – ' (whatever events were happening on the Saturday). Life would return to normal for the next three weeks, apart from the clinic visits for the injection of the drug as an outpatient. These visits were usually on a Wednesday. We would set off early, have her check-up and injection and generally she would be back in Paddock Wood in time for afternoon school. This procedure went on for nearly twelve months, and the only schooling that Rachel missed was two days every three weeks. She was adamant that this treatment was not going to interfere with anything unless it was absolutely necessary.

During the year of chemotherapy Rachel was always given Maxolon, an anti-sickness drug. It eased the vomiting a little and on one occasion, when she had been particularly sick, the day was coming to an end and she had another injection. The nurse told me that she probably wouldn't need any further doses as the vomiting was beginning to wane. After the nurse had gone, Rach, Gran and I resumed the game we were playing, but when it came to Rachel's turn there was no reaction. I spoke to her and there was no reply. I looked up at her and was faced with a horrifying sight. Rachel was sitting in bed with just the whites of her eyes showing and a stream of dribble running from her mouth. At first I thought she was up to her old tricks again and told her not to do that with her eyes as she would strain the muscles. No response. 'Stop mucking about, Rachel.' No response. Gran told her to stop it. No response. Panic set in and I ran up the corridor for the nurse who looked at Rachel and said there was nothing to worry about, she would be all right. I was annoyed and said, 'For goodness' sake, look at her, she's far from all right.' She told me she would bleep the doctor. Meanwhile Pete's Mum was trying to get Rachel to swallow by massaging her neck. Again there was no response.

When the doctor arrived he explained that it was a side-effect of the Maxolon that could happen at any time and gradually she would return to normal. We had never been told that Maxolon could produce side-effects and we could not comprehend how she would ever be all right again; her irises had completely disappeared and she was dribbling uncontrollably. It was very frightening. Peter arrived in the middle of all this confusion. Peter has always had a calming effect on me and again told me to trust the doctors. 'If there's nothing to worry about, then don't worry,' he said.

After about two hours Rachel's eyes began to come down from the top of her head for short spells, then disappear again. After about three hours she was back to normal, thinking the whole thing was extremely amusing. She described it to us as being trapped inside her own body: she could hear and understand everything we said to her, but she couldn't respond. She thought it was hilarious hearing us going bananas, but she couldn't tell us she was OK. She looked as though she had suffered some sort of brain damage, but that was because she couldn't make anything work. She said the only discomfort she felt was that her eyes were sore. Rachel thought the funniest thing about this particular episode was Gran trying to coax her to swallow by massaging her throat: 'That's what you used to do to Barney [her dog] to make him swallow his pills.' The rest of us felt we had aged twenty years, although, thank goodness, Rach was none the worse for wear. After that I asked for her never to have Maxolon again. The doctors understood my concern, saying it would probably never happen again, but they readily agreed not to take that chance.

Rachel never lost her sense of humour and fun. During one of our stays in hospital, Andy Stockdale, the chemo-therapy registrar, had asked an eminent surgeon, Mr Paul Acroath, to examine Rachel's leg in case surgery was required at a later date. He told Rachel that Mr Acroath was a very important and busy man. A mischievous twinkle came into her eyes and I wondered what she was thinking. The morn-ing ward round began, everything was ship-shape and Mr Acroath, his students and colleagues somehow all squeezed in to Rachel's little cubicle. The patient was lying very still and quiet with the covers under her chin. Mr Acroath began to talk to his colleagues in his own medical way and asked the patient if he might examine her leg. The bed covers erupted and out bounced Rachel exclaiming, 'Boo!' She had put the head of a Girl's World make-up bust on her pillow and hidden herself under the covers. Mr Acroath's team stifled sniggers. Andy went white. I think Mr Acroath was also quite amused, in his own way.

On another occasion Rachel was in hospital for one of her weekly injections and we were waiting in our cubicle for Andy. Rach had some sweets which looked just like eyeballs. She placed them in her eye-sockets and screwed up her face to hold them in. Then she called for Andy, saying her eyes were hurting her. Andy came in and burst out laughing, and so did the nurses.

Towards the end of the twelve months, Rachel had to have radiotherapy treatment to her tibia. For twenty days through December we had to attend the Westminster Hospital for a five-minute dose of radiotherapy. We were offered a bed, as the doctors said that the radiotherapy might make Rachel tired, but Rachel would not hear of it. 'I shall become a commuter,' she said. 'I don't want to miss school.' The doctors agreed that if she felt she could cope, she could travel to London each day for her treatment, and that is what we did. We had our appointments fitted as much as possible around Rachel's school days and she coped as she always did, with no problems. The hospital was wonderful and got us in and out as quickly as possible. She had no ill-effects from the radiotherapy, but by the weekend she was grateful for the rest from travelling. During the approach to Christmas she took charge of decorating the radiotherapy department on odd occasions when we had to wait for a while for our turn. She always used every minute of her time. Whenever we went for appointments or check-ups Rachel was allowed to go behind the reception desk where she would book in other patients for further appointments and answer the phone with the receptionists looking on. Everyone treated her so well, and she became everyone's friend.

When the last chemotherapy was due the doctors said they would remove the Hickman Line before we went home which would free Rachel completely. She wanted a general anaesthetic to remove the line, but the doctors said they could pull it out very quickly with a local, which would mean she could go home as usual. After much persuasion, Rachel agreed. We were in Rachel's cubicle and I was reading to her when she suddenly announced that her bed was wet. Not believing her, expecting one of her tricks, I pulled back the covers to find the Hickman Line lying on her bed, pumping out saline. The doctor was amazed and suggested that Rachel had helped it out in some way, especially as she knew it was going to be removed. But I had been with her all the time and I knew she had not done anything to it. It was lovely to see the relief on her face when she realized that she had got rid of it on her own. She skipped around the cubicle singing, 'I free, I'm free!' I sometimes wonder if her strong-mindedness had willed that line out of her body. She was a very determined young lady who knew what she did and didn't want.

As the year drew to a close she had a scan which came back even better than the last. There had been a steady improvement on each scan, and the last one came back looking normal. We were all so excited and the doctors were delighted with the way things were going. They seemed to have put Rachel's cancer into remission with the last chemotherapy treatment. With a normal-looking scan, all seemed wonderful again. The doctors said they would be keeping a watchful eye on Rachel, with regular scans and check-ups. I remember thinking, 'We are going to win this one.'

Rachel went off to school full of her news and told everyone she was better now and would soon be able to go horse-riding again and swimming. She had been unable to go swimming for the last year because of the Hickman Line. We tried once, with the permission of the doctors, fixing a special dressing over the area where the Hickman Line entered her body. After only a few minutes in the pool it started to unstick so she was whipped out of the water and quickly showered and dressed. Despite our quick reactions and efforts, an infection ensued and put her in hospital for a week. It was so frustrating – even the smallest treat we tried to give her she had to pay dearly for. Needless to say, we didn't try that again.

CHAPTER FOUR

WITH THE CHEMO FINISHED and the Hickman Line gone
we were really free. Rachel went swimming as soon as the
wound had healed, which was only a week or so later, and
we started to swim as a family again every weekend. It was
overwhelming to see her able to join in and be so carefree;
she had certainly earned her freedom after all she had been
through. We also planned a holiday as we felt we all needed
a rest and a change of scenery, especially Rachel. We had
planned to go to Switzerland the previous year, but Rachel's
treatment had made that impossible. Now we decided that
Switzerland would be the ideal place for a carefree, happy
holiday.

We went to Grindelwald where we had rented a chalet
facing the north face of the Eiger. It was beautiful. We
arrived in glorious sunshine and the spring flowers were out
in abundance. We didn't have a care in the world. We were
all so happy and excited, and determined we were going to
enjoy this holiday after the horrors of the last year, no matter
what. We walked to various places around Grindelwald and
took train trips to all the little hamlets scattered round about.
We went on chair lifts and boat trips and then one morning
we woke up to about eight inches of snow. It was like seeing
everything for the first time again, for it was quite different
in the snow. The girls had a lovely time playing with snow-

balls. We took a trip up the mountain in the train and the higher we got, the deeper the snow. It was like having a winter and summer holiday all in one. We came home rested and refreshed, ready to take on the world.

While we were in Switzerland Rachel had decided to dispose of her wig. Although her hair was extremely short, at that time it was very trendy, so she felt she was the height of fashion. Once the wig had gone she felt just the same as everyone else. No more worries about windy days.

Her hair grew very quickly, and it was absolutely beautiful. The colour was the same and the texture was much improved; it became very shiny and had a slight curl. She was delighted with herself, and so were we.

We had put our house up for sale before we left for our holiday, just to test the market, and by the time we got back we had a buyer. Almost at once we found a house in the area that we all liked. It was much bigger than our present house, but with the girls growing up we felt we needed to spread our wings a bit. The formalities of sale and purchase went without a hitch, and soon we were all busy turning out and packing up.

Rachel and Katy designed their rooms and chose new colour schemes before we had even signed the contracts. The thought of moving the girls' rooms, especially Rachel's, from one house to another filled us with apprehension. It was a standing joke within the family that if anything went missing, it was sure to be found in Rachel's room, usually under her bed. It was Peter who proclaimed he had solved the mystery of the Bermuda Triangle. When Rachel said excitedly 'Where Dad?', he replied, 'It's under your bed!'

On moving day the girls went off to school feeling very excited. We kissed them goodbye and reminded them for the thousandth time not to forget to come home to our new address. After school they were quite indignant that everything was not yet in its right place. They set to and helped us to finish the essential jobs. Here we were in our new home, a happy little family of four who had come through a rough time and were now looking forward to a fresh start without worries about illness and hospitals.

In July Rachel asked if she could go to Guide Camp and although I was a little worried about her going away without us, we decided that she must be allowed to be like any other little girl. I had become a little over-protective, but Peter helped me a lot by talking things through in his usual logical manner. Rachel's guider was very understanding and we armed her with lots of emergency telephone numbers and detailed instructions about what Rachel could and couldn't do (she was inclined to say she could do things that she knew she must not – but who could blame her after a year of being tied down?).

We were worried all the time Rachel was away, but she had a lovely time and came home full of what they had been doing and places she had visited. She told us how she had managed to hit her bad leg with a mallet while putting up the tent. My heart missed a beat, but she appeared no worse for it.

In August we were due for a scan. Rachel appeared to be so well that we weren't too worried, although we never slept well the night before a scan. The hospital had taught me what to look for and after so many scans I was quite good at interpreting the pictures that came up on the screen. So was Rachel. They always gave her a complete body scan and when we got to the left tibia a very slight shadow appeared. My heart sank and Rachel began to cry, but we decided it couldn't be anything to worry about as she had had no pain. Even so, the worries came flooding back.

The doctors looked at the scans and listened to our worries, but convinced us we were worrying about nothing; they thought it was a healing process that the scan had picked up. Sometimes radiotherapy treatment causes the scan to pick up 'hot spots', as the treatment causes damage to the bone as well as to the tumour. This sounded reasonable, so our worries were put in the background. They were doctors and understood these things far more than we did. They hadn't let us down yet, and we had complete faith in them. The difference in Rachel was astounding, so they must have got it right. We went home again and back to our lives, perhaps not totally relaxed but hopeful.

Rachel awoke on the morning of 3 September crying with the pain in her leg. All those niggles in the back of my mind came racing to the fore and I rang the Westminster Hospital immediately. They invited me to take Rachel to them. The poor little soul cried all the way to London on the train, both from fright and the pain. When we arrived the doctors did all the usual tests and everything came back looking good. They took me to one side and said they thought that seeing the last scan might have upset Rachel and that the pain she was now experiencing could be due to anxiety. It seemed a reasonable assumption because on seeing her X-rays and hearing that all the other tests were satisfactory she seemed far more relaxed and the pain subsided. The doctors said they were not at all worried about Rachel, but if at any time I felt anxious about her I was to ring and they would see us.

We returned home and everything settled down again, except that from time to time Rachel would become quiet and tearful. When I questioned her she would assure me she was in no pain but that she just felt like crying, so we would sit down and have a talk about things. Sometimes we would both have a good cry, then we would blow our noses, wipe away each other's tears and laugh at ourselves for being wallies. I had a chat with my own GP about Rachel and he talked with her from time to time. He too felt that the emotions of her horrendous year of treatment had to be expressed at some time, and that now that things had calmed down, she had time to think about all she had gone through and to feel a little sorry for herself. If she wanted to cry, we should encourage her to, and talk about all the things that worried her. This we did, and her periods of being down became less frequent.

Rachel still experienced odd bouts of pain in her leg, which I always told the hospital about. On 31 October we were sent to see Mr Acroath, the orthopaedic surgeon Rachel had seen before in the Westminster. He had been kept up-to-date on her progress and he wanted to be sure that the 'hot spots' seen on the scan were in fact a healing process and not tumour regrowth. He suggested that we should have another bone biopsy as this was the only sure way of knowing. We asked him about the options available if it was tumour regrowth. His answer was a mid-thigh amputation if the rest of her body was clear. This was all that could be done as she had had all the chemotherapy and radiotherapy that she could have. We had been offered an amputation before and refused, hoping that the drugs could save her leg. Now if we were faced with the choice of her leg or her life, there would be no contest.

All our hopes now were pinned on the 'hot spots' showing radiotherapy damage and nothing more sinister.

CHAPTER FIVE

ON 5 DECEMBER we were admitted to Westminster Children's Hospital for the biopsy. Rachel was terrified at the prospect of another operation – and who could blame her? She went to the theatre, calling me not to leave her. I went as far as the theatre staff would allow (because of the risk of infection) but then she was on her own. I hated to leave her when she needed me most and blocked my ears so that I couldn't hear her calling me. I went back to the ward and waited.

After what seemed like hours they said Rachel was ready to come back to the ward so I went down with the nurse and picked her up from theatre. She was her usual noisy self, telling the theatre staff she hated them, and that her leg hurt, and that she wanted her Mum. That was always a welcome noise because then I knew she was all right. I always had a secret fear that she would not come out of the anaesthetic. Once I heard her yelling I could cope, because I knew she was conscious.

We were told she had to stay in hospital for four or five days. During that time the hospital held a Christmas party for current and past patients. Rachel had received an invitation weeks before, and we had accepted, not dreaming that she would be an inpatient at the time.

On the afternoon of the party Rachel plonked herself into

a wheelchair with her leg elevated and got Katy to take her downstairs to the party; she had offered to help distribute food to the children. While this was going on, one of the doctors came to see her on the ward and was a little bewildered when she could not be found. Apparently she should have been on complete bed-rest, but someone had forgotten to tell the ward sister and she had allowed Rachel to go to the party. When we found Rachel she had her wheelchair piled high with goodies for the other children and was happily ordering her sister around to enable her to make her deliveries.

A couple of days later we were allowed home again, armed with painkillers. The result of the biopsy would take about ten days to come through.

After the bone biopsy, Rachel experienced more pain and discomfort. Although the doctors had had to operate to find out what was going on, the intrusion seemed to make things worse. She was constantly on painkillers and had lost her usual sparkle. I was able to get a wheelchair on loan from our local health centre, but Rachel did not take kindly to it. She found she could not walk as far as before without the pain getting really bad, so I said to her, 'You either spend all your time at home, or ignore the stares you get from people,' (because people do stare and it's very upsetting for the person in the wheelchair) 'and treat them with the contempt they deserve.'

Rachel decided she would grin and bear it, and so I would take her for walks in the afternoon which at least gave her some fresh air and something else to think about. At weekends, of course, it was much easier because Peter was at home, and we could go in the car, with the wheelchair in the back, to the seaside or to the market. Rachel enjoyed these outings; she felt useful when we went to the market because she could carry all the shopping for us on her knees. Peter then pushed the wheelchair which was heavy and cumbersome, but he would do wheelies and skids with it and Rachel would shriek with laughter. During the week she would say, 'Go on, Mum, do a wheelie like Dad does.' 'You must be joking!' I would answer. 'Roll on the weekend, then!' was always her reply.

On 19 December we went to see Mr Acroath. As soon as we saw his face we knew he had bad news for us. He told us that Rachel's tumour had returned and she needed an amputation, and that we should go home and have a nice Christmas and he would see us in the New Year.

I was livid. How could we have a nice Christmas with this hanging over us? If it had to be done I wanted to get on with it. If the cancer was active again, surely time was of the essence – we didn't want it to spread any further. Mr Acroath said that two weeks were not going to make any difference and insisted that we should go home and forget about it until the New Year.

We left Mr Acroath's office with that familiar numb feeling and for the first time I felt as if everything was falling apart. I was very angry and bitter. How could we have a nice Christmas? Rachel was constantly down and in very bad pain, we had just been told her cancer had regrown. I wanted something done immediately. I ranted and raved about everything winding down for Christmas in the hospital, about being caught up in the system, and that Rachel should be treated immediately. Rachel had one of the fastest-growing cancers known and we were wasting precious time, trying to have a nice Christmas while the tumour was growing unchecked. I wanted Christmas postponed. I asked the doctors to get on with what had to be done, and then we could have Christmas later. The only important thing to us was to get Rachel better, or at least out of immediate danger. We didn't care about Christmas.

The doctors listened but restated what we had already been told, that two weeks would make no difference, and that it was important to have Christmas and enjoy ourselves, rather than have Rachel in hospital at such a special time of the year. But they didn't have to sit and watch her suffer, knowing there was nothing to do until it was time for the next painkiller when she would have a short time pain-free. Then it would get worse. We were constantly looking at our watches, wishing the time away until we could give her more drugs to make her comfortable. I felt utterly helpless.

We took Rachel home and we had Christmas. She did enjoy the pain-free time, and even when she was in pain she didn't complain. She just sat in a chair and watched the rest of the family, joining in when her pain allowed. We went to Peter's Mum and Dad's for Christmas Day. Peter's sisters came with their husbands and children, as did his Aunty Kathleen and her husband Uncle Chas. Aunty Kathleen was dying of cancer and we all knew it was going to be her last Christmas.

No one knew it was to be our Rachel's last Christmas. Now, after all that has happened, I can see it was important for Rachel to have Christmas at home with all her family around her. Perhaps the doctors, by insisting that we took her home, were telling us that this was her last Christmas, but we hadn't wanted to pick up on those kind of thoughts at that time. We were all trying to stay positive and maybe the doctors hadn't wanted to destroy that.

On Boxing Day we went to my sister's with my Mum and Dad. There were also some family friends there and we had a lovely day. Again Rachel was only able to join in when her pain allowed, but she said she had enjoyed herself, and cuddled up to her Granddad when the pain got bad to play 'I spy' or something similar.

After Christmas the days dragged on to New Year. We all said, this year our luck has got to change. Perhaps Rachel will get better. On 5 January we were admitted to the Westminster Hospital for the amputation of Rachel's tibia. First she had to have a complete body and lung scan to make sure the rest of her body was clear of cancer. The CT scan of Rachel's lungs showed that they were clear. First hurdle over and a sigh of relief. The next day came the gamma scan of Rachel's whole body (this is a bone scan). That night I went home for a break and told Rachel I would see her in the morning. She was quite happy for me to go home as she knew that she had had all the tests done and was just waiting for the results.

The next day, as Peter and I walked into the hospital, we met one of the doctors in the corridor. I took one look at his face and knew something was wrong. We asked if he had Rachel's results. He said he was sorry to tell us they had found more tumour in Rachel's spine. The next thing I remember we were in the consulting rooms with the doctor and a nurse, and he was telling us that an amputation was out of the question as Rachel had tumour elsewhere. He had nothing else to offer us surgically. He said there was a meeting that afternoon with the chemo and orthopaedic teams which we should attend. He then left us alone to pull ourselves together, and to find Rachel who was totally unaware of this new development.

We went on to the ward to find Rachel and we carried on as usual, except to say that we had to go to a meeting to see the doctors that afternoon for results. She wasn't very interested in all that, as she had other things on her mind. She told us excitedly that she had been asked to do a radio

39

interview for Radio 4's 'Woman's Hour' that afternoon about play workers within the hospital. She was far too preoccupied with that to worry about doctors' meetings. This proved to be a welcome distraction for us all, and we chatted about what she would say.

Rachel's father John, Peter and I went off for our meeting and left a very excited young lady on the ward waiting to make her debut on the radio. We all felt hopeless, tense and nervous. When we had settled down Mr Hanam, the chemotherapy consultant, introduced us to Professor Barrett, a haematologist who had devised a new drug called BCNU. He explained that this drug had been tried and tested and that the idea was to remove part of Rachel's bone marrow and freeze it, once it had been tested and found to be clear of cancer cells. Then she would be given this new drug which would kill everything in her body; good and bad, her immune system would be completely wiped out, leaving her wide open to any infection going. After three days she would be given her bone marrow back again and then she would have to wait for her bone marrow to build a new immune system. The theory was that both good and bad cells in Rachel's body would be killed and the clean bone marrow would start a new, fresh, clean system. If this treatment cured the tumour in her spine, then after a time her leg could be amputated. There were no guarantees, but then we had never had any before, so we were not surprised there was none now.

The treatment sounded terrifying, but at the same time it was wonderful to think that there was at least something else we could try. I had been so afraid that they were going to say they could do no more and send Rachel home to die. We went in feeling hopeless, and came out scared to death at the prospect of what we were going to put Rachel through. We were trapped. What could we do? We had to go forward and be positive, and at least we had a chance this way. Heads spinning, we left the doctors and after some discussion we decided that we had to give Rachel that chance. If we did nothing, she would die. She could die while she was having the treatment, but at least we were giving her a chance. The doctors had told us that we should look on the treatment as buying time for her; a complete cure would be a bonus.

The next step was to tell Rachel. We had always told her the truth and explained everything honestly, but after talking it through, we felt that she should not be told about her cancer spreading. Her morale was too low after so many weeks in pain. If we told her that she had tumours elsewhere, she might just give up and say what's the point? So we lied to Rachel for the first time.

We told her an amputation could not be done. Of course she wanted to know why. We told her that her leg was too angry to amputate just now and that the doctors wanted to give her these drugs to calm it down. If all went well, the leg would then be amputated. At first she said she would take no more drugs. We couldn't blame her for reacting this way – we didn't have to experience the feelings she had – she was frightened. She cried and cried, and kept saying No, No, No, but we explained that if we did nothing she would surely die. It is a terrible choice to have to make, a terrible thing to have to explain to your child. I felt so cruel. I wished so many times that I could have had the treatment for her; I would have done anything to have her well. We told her the truth about the treatment, and gave her every detail about the effects of the drug and about the fact that she could die from the treatment itself. We hid only the fact that her tumour had spread.

We talked for a long time and then in her usual way she said, 'Let's forget it now and do something else.' She changed the subject and told us all about her radio interview and which day it would be transmitted so that we could note it in our diaries and tell everyone to listen out for her. Later a staff nurse came in and told us that as we had so much to think about we should go home for the weekend.

This perked Rachel up no end and in a flash we were packed up and ready to go, but we left a lot of her things at the hospital. After more discussion at home Rachel decided that if she wanted to live, then she had to go ahead. When it comes to the crunch, you don't have a choice at all because no one wants to die. Where Rachel got her courage and strength from I do not know. I have always been proud of my children, but never so much as then. If I had been given that choice for myself, I'm sure I would have given up, but Rachel was a fighter. We had a lovely weekend, except for the times when her pain increased before it was time for the next pill. Then the weather changed.

With the snow came worries about travelling back to London. The doctors had said they would get everything organized and let us know when they were ready. Rachel was delighted and said she didn't care how long they took; she just wanted to stay at home. We, however, were eager to press on because we didn't want her to be in pain any longer, or for the cancer to spread. When Rachel's pain was bad she would say, 'I can't wait for this treatment. This pain is driving me mad.' But after a painkiller she would change her mind again, because whenever she was pain-free she could cope, as could we all. It was like a see-saw. We knew that, if left, her pain would get worse and worse and the painkillers would have to be stronger and stronger until she would be put on morphine and not know whether it was day or night. That we could not bear, Rachel was too special for that.

The snow got worse and worse, and one morning we had a phone call from John saying that he had got some sledges for the children and did we think Rachel was up to going out in the snow on one. She was pretty immobile at this time and felt she could not cope walking in such deep snow, so we invited him to come around to our house and we all took turns pulling Rachel around the back garden. It was so special to hear her shrieks of laughter and we took some of the happiest photographs we have of her. All too soon her pain returned and our garden games came to an end, but at least she had had a little time out in the snow enjoying herself.

A few days later we had notification from London that they were ready for us. Panic set in because the trains were at a standstill and car travel was impossible. Now what would we do? Rachel belonged to the Red Cross youth movement and they kindly said they would take us in their ambulance, so on 15 January we set off for Westminster Children's Hospital in appalling weather and road conditions, armed with flasks of coffee and packets of sandwiches, sleeping bags and shovels. Rachel knew all the volunteers who took us, and we began to chat about all the things the Red Cross group had been doing to help others during the bad weather. The boys said how useful a radio in the ambulance would be as they had to keep returning to base to find out their next assignment. Indeed, our own base at Paddock Wood had no idea whether we were getting through or not. The only way we could let them know was by telephone. We eventually arrived safely at Westminster Children's Hospital, thanked the boys for all their help and wished them a safe journey back. We entered the hospital half relieved that we could finally get on with making Rachel better, and half scared out of our wits at the thought of what was to come. We went on to the ward and received the usual warm greetings, and settled down to see doctors and start the unending tests.

While we were waiting Rachel asked her Dad and me if we could buy the Red Cross a radio for their ambulance as a present for taking us all to the hospital. We explained that we would love to be able to do that, but that we could not afford it. We said that we would give them a donation for their funds.

Soon the doctors arrived and explained what was going to happen first. Rachel had to have an operation to have another Hickman Line inserted so that they could give her the drugs and back-up medication without any discomfort. While they had her out, they were going to remove about a pint of her bone marrow. It would be checked for cancer cells and if it was all clear it would then be frozen, ready to give back to her when she had had the BCNU drug.

When the time came for her operation, Rachel was terrified. As usual, the pre-med was given and Rachel was nice and relaxed, but as soon as she heard the trolley arrive and saw the men in their theatre clothes, she would fight the pre-med and begin to get upset. I went down to the theatre with her as I always did, and this time we had an anaesthetist who didn't mind mums being with the children while they were put under.

The anaesthetist was unable to find a vein in Rachel's hand. Then he tried her wrist. The only decent vein he could find was in Rachel's arm, but the surgeons had said they wanted that left free because she would have to come out of theatre on a drip. They decided Rachel would have to have gas. By this time she was distraught from being pricked so often and I was finding it very hard to keep control of myself. She refused to take the mask with the gas, and so the anaesthetist had to try and get her under by waving the tube carrying the gas under her nose. It didn't have much effect because Rachel was so upset. The surgeons were becoming restless and wanted to proceed. Rachel fought all the time and I began to reach the point where I couldn't bear this man to do all these things to my child. I asked him to leave her alone. He assured me Rachel would remember none of what was going on and gradually she began to fall asleep.

When I was sure she was asleep I left her. They took my daughter into theatre. I was shaking from head to foot when I rejoined Peter outside, and the poor man was in just as bad shape. He had heard Rachel crying and screaming, and he had no idea what was going on. I don't know which was worse.

We went back on the ward and waited. It seemed such a long time, but after about an hour the call came to go and pick up Rachel from theatre. As usual, I could hear her calling me and telling the theatre staff to go away and get her Mum. What a welcome sound! We got Rachel back to the ward and put her into bed and she soon settled down for a good long sleep. When she woke up she was very sore; her back was a mass of needle marks where they had taken her marrow. Peter and I had decided not to make any comment about the incident in the ante-room, but Rachel broached the subject and related exactly what had happened. She had total recall of the incident. So much for the anaesthetist – what did he know? The only thing she didn't remember was that I was, in fact, there by her side. That chain of events stayed with Rachel vividly, so much so that she began to worry about the next visit to theatre. I knew how she felt; that experience was something I will always remember. We calmed her down and told her not to worry about the future, that it was all over for now and she must try to forget about it. In a few days the needle marks turned yellow and blue with bruising and it brought tears to our eyes to see what had been done to her. The results from the bone marrow tests were good, it was clear of any cancer cells and had been frozen. The next step was to give her the BCNU drug. The ward that we were going to for Rachel's treatment was found to have a bug on it. It would not have affected most children but it could have killed Rachel because once her immune system had been wiped out she would have no reserves to fight anything; even a common cold could be extremely dangerous, if not fatal to her. A safe ward was found in the Charing Cross Hospital at Hammersmith and we were duly transferred there on 20 January, initially to Bristol Ward.

We were told the treatment would take about four weeks, but it turned out to be nearer eight. When we first arrived at Bristol Ward we were apprehensive enough about the treatment without having to get used to a new team of doctors and nurses, but we needn't have worried. They were a superb team and became our friends as well, in some cases close friends. They were confronted with a very frightened and tearful little girl in a wheelchair with a very swollen and painful leg and a Mum who was also bewildered and frightened. Within a couple of hours we had been shown the room that was to become Rachel's home for the weeks ahead.

We had been told that a few days after Rachel had the drug her white cell count would gradually go down until it finally disappeared. She would become neutropaenic (no immune system) and we would have to reverse barrier nurse her and it was then that it was most dangerous. The reverse barrier nursing would be carried on until her cell counts came back up, which would mean she could then cope with any infection that might come her way.

They explained to us in great detail what would happen to Rachel when the drug was given. We were told she would vomit almost immediately; her skin would flush, reddening as it does after strenuous exercise; she would appear to sweat profusely and her eyes would water as if she were crying. It all sounded terrifying, but Rachel said, 'Let's get it over with and stop talking about it.'

Once we had settled in, every test imaginable was carried out on Rachel to make sure she was germ-free before we started. A date for administering the drug was set: 27 January. When we arrived at the Charing Cross I had told the nurses that I wanted to move into the hospital with Rachel. They said there was no problem as mothers were accommodated. We had mattresses given to us and at night we would take them down to the playroom and make our beds. We were given bags to put our linen in and if there were several of us each would put her name and child's name at the bottom of the mattress so that if your child wanted you in the night, the nurses would creep in to wake the mother concerned. It was just like a dormitory. The nurses had so much to do but they always found time for the mums and did their best to help us. In the evenings when the children were asleep the mums would congregate and swap notes about their children and ailments. We would console each other on bad days and be happy with each other on good days. Some children were seriously ill and some were not, but there was always some-one to pass the long lonely evenings with and it was a comfort in a funny sort of way to talk to someone with similar problems. We helped each other.

CHAPTER SIX

JANUARY 27TH DAWNED. After a very restless night, I packed up my bed and went to find Rachel. She was feeling the same – terrified of what the day was going to entail. We sat quietly on our own and talked it through, cried a little and had a cuddle. Then we dried each other's tears and said, 'This time tomorrow it will all be over, so let's get cracking.'

I was not supposed to stay with Rachel while they administered the drugs, as I was told the fumes would give me a terrible headache. I had to choose whether to be with her while she had the drug, or to sit with her afterwards once the air had had a chance to clear. Another decision. Rachel and I discussed it. The walls were mainly glass and so she said she wanted me to stand by the window so she could see me and I could see her, and then she wanted me to go and sit with her after they had finished. So that is what I did. The nurses and doctors were gowned and masked, gloved and goggled (to protect their eyes from the fumes). It was intimidating to watch them all squeezing into her little room armed with syringes and drugs. Rachel had asked to be dosed with lorazepam as she had before, but unfortunately it didn't seem to have much effect. I think she was so frightened that nothing would have calmed her. As they began to draw up the drugs and prepare themselves, Rachel became more and more agitated. She was trying so hard to go to sleep and block them out, but she couldn't. Panic set in. She did not want to witness what they were doing to her. After what seemed an eternity someone decided to give her some valium, and gradually she became drowsy and drifted off to sleep. What relief I felt as I watched her first calm then finally relax and sleep. I didn't want her to be aware of too much that was happening.

At last they began. Mixed feelings of 'Hurry up and get it done' and 'Please stop, I'm not sure', were surging through me. It was my turn to panic. Being on the other side of the glass and feeling utterly helpless and useless, I watched as the BCNU was slowly injected into Rachel's Hickman Line. I watched Rachel and I watched the doctors, praying that this time it was going to work and give my little one what other people took for granted – a fit and healthy life, for however long. As the doctors had warned me, Rachel started to vomit, but she was so drugged that she wasn't aware of it. Then I began to worry that she might choke, but the nurses were watching her very carefully and she was turned on her side and her mouth cleared quickly and efficiently. After about half an hour it was finished and the doctors prepared to leave the cubicle. When they came out they said to wait for about ten minutes for the air to clear (they had opened all the windows) and then I could sit with her.

I gowned and masked up and went in to Rachel. By now she was slowly turning very red and her eyes were beginning to run, just as I had been warned, but she was sound asleep. A trained nurse stayed with me and monitored Rachel's every move. She explained to me that the effects would last for about four hours, but that Rachel would probably not wake up until the next morning. Even then, she would be confused, but I was not to worry as that was to be expected because the drugs to relax her had been given in fairly high doses.

We sat with Rachel all morning and then the nurses changed shifts. After they had done a report and felt confident that Rachel would be all right, they left me with her and told me to buzz for them if I was worried about anything. At about 3.30 P.M. Rachel was sick again, but this time she didn't go straight back to sleep. She began to talk to me, and asked what the time was and could she have a drink. I buzzed for a nurse who came immediately. She called the sister who said Rachel shouldn't even be awake let alone wanting a drink. She gowned and masked up and came in. She was amazed at just how awake Rachel was. She told her she could wet her lips holding a glass, but she must not drink. This Rachel did and as Sister Jane and I were talking, I turned back to look at Rachel who was holding the glass to her mouth. I reminded her she must not drink. 'Don't worry, Mum,' she said. 'My lips are just absorbing the moisture.' I looked at Jane and said, 'And that's confused?' Jane was also surprised by Rachel's awareness. Within half an hour she asked for the television to be put on because she didn't want to miss the children's programmes.

Peter arrived shortly afterwards, having had reports on the telephone during the day. He gowned and masked up and when he came in he said, 'Hello, Mouse [his nickname for her], how you doing?' 'OK, thanks, Dad. You do look a wally dressed like that!' Apart from a sore tummy, Rachel seemed fine. Peter and I were so relieved that it was all over. The next time she saw Professor Barrett, Rachel told him, 'It wasn't that bad, but I'm not having any more, OK?' He smiled at her and told her what a good patient she had been.

Rachel started liquids that evening. When asked later if she had any pain and would she like a painkiller, she replied,

'No pain, that BCNU's good stuff.' Rachel never had to take another painkiller. It was remarkable. Pete went home and I went to bed and Rachel was already sleeping peacefully. After a very hard day, it was lovely to watch her.

Next morning Rachel woke up feeling a bit fragile, but we persuaded her to try and eat a little breakfast to take the soreness away. As always she was willing to try, and after her breakfast she didn't look back. She was eating crisps and drinking Coke by lunchtime. She had to have her blood taken every day so that they could monitor the counts – white count, red count, platelets, electrolytes, neutrophils etcetera. The blood is made up of many different components and each had to be monitored. Pete and I understood some of the more common counts but it became very complicated and hard for us to follow without medical knowledge, so we had to put our trust in the doctors once again.

The white count disappeared completely after about five days, but before that happened Sister Jane started us on reverse barrier nursing. As she said, we were bound to make mistakes at first and didn't want any mistakes made when it was vital to Rachel's safety. This is what had to be done: dispray (a disinfectant spray) everything that went into her room; change her bed linen every day; damp dust her room twice a day; disinfect the floor twice a day; put all her eating utensils in Milton solution; microwave all her food; change her soap every other day; use clean flannels every day. She was not allowed to wear anything twice without it being washed; she had to drink sterilized water; Coke or any other bottled drink had to be changed daily; if she wanted bread it had to be a slice taken from the middle of a new loaf.

There were no visitors except for Peter, myself and John. They rigged up an intercom for her so she could talk to people through the glass. When Rachel and I talked about the treatment later, she said the worst bit for her had been being shut in the room all the time, and not being able to kiss and cuddle us properly. I had to agree with her, I could kiss her on her head and put an arm round her, but it was like cuddling from a distance. As with everything else, she understood that it was for the best, just in case we had any germs around that we didn't know about.

Eventually Rachel was ready to have her bone marrow returned to her and a doctor brought it from the Westminster Hospital in a cannister. Rachel wasn't perturbed because the doctors had told her it would be just like having a saline drip, something she had become quite used to. The doctors and nurses masked and gowned up and went in with Rachel, and I took up my familiar position on the other side of the glass. It looked like a scene from a space programme. The marrow had been stored in liquid nitrogen and when they opened it up a white mist came out of the cannister. The doctor then filled a basin with water into which he placed the bags containing the bone marrow. Crackling and vapour filled the room. The doctor wore goggles and gauntlet gloves and soon there was quite a crowd of other nurses and doctors on the outside with me, trying to get a glimpse of what was going on. Rachel took it all in her stride and was laughing and joking with them while they prepared the marrow to go in the drip. The smell was disgusting, like stale cabbage water. It hung around the ward all day and most of the next. This part of the treatment was quite easy to cope with and once the doctors had finished rigging up the drip I was allowed in again.

Rachel and I passed a usual sort of day, watching the video, playing games, writing letters and eating and drinking. Rachel's count was still going down and within a couple of days had completely disappeared. Now it was for real with the reverse barrier nursing and we all became neurotic about germs and infections. Our hands were sore from continuous washings and we would spray everything in sight. Rachel found all this highly amusing; because she was quite well in herself and pain-free, she was full of beans. Her old sparkle had come back. The tricks started again and her appetite was back with gusto. Life didn't seem too bad. We felt things would improve again; if we could just get her counts up and keep her out of danger from infections, perhaps we would be in with a chance.

CHAPTER SEVEN

DAYS PASSED with the usual routine of reverse barrier nursing care, playing games and just generally passing the time. Some days were better than others. Sometimes Rachel would cry, sad, just because she wanted to go home. She missed her sister and family and friends and of course her freedom. At least I could go out on to the ward, or go to the shops, and just have a break, but Rachel couldn't leave her cubicle. Sometimes it all became too much, which was quite understandable. But for most of the time she was happy and mischievous.

On 13 February, seventeen days after the drug had been introduced to her, her count began to appear. Great celebrations! Rachel had a white cell count of .06 which was very dangerously low, but at least it was showing signs that the bone marrow was working. It felt like nothing short of a miracle. As soon as she heard the news she was asking, 'How much longer before I can go on the ward?' 'How much longer before I can go home?' The doctors said that her count had to be .05 neutrophils − cells in the blood that protect us naturally from infections − and they could not say how long this would take. Everyone's body repairs itself at different rates. So Rachel continued with her caged-up days without complaint.

One of Rachel's talents was for drawing, and with all these

days in such a confined space she produced some of the best drawings I had ever seen her do. Everyone, doctors, nurses and even other parents, came to look through the window at her drawings, and all began asking her to do something special for them. She was soon inundated with requests, and devised a scheme to avoid disappointing anyone. She would do a drawing and then her Dad would photocopy it. Most of her pictures were of animals and birds, and so Rachel was able to give copies to everyone who wanted them.

At times it was hard to find something different to do to make the time go faster. One day was especially memorable. Cancer Research had brought a multitude of balloons filled with helium for the children. At first they were a novelty, silver and pink with cute little creatures and trendy slogans on them, but the children soon tired of them, so Rachel asked if they could all be put in her room. The nurses, bless them, sprayed them all with dispray to keep out the germs and they were duly sent in. Rachel spent the morning writing begging notes, asking for money for the Bristol Ward at the Charing Cross Hospital and I spent the morning tying them to the balloons and then releasing them from the window. Sadly no one replied, but it passed the time and gave us something to look forward to for a few days, hoping someone rich would find one and donate a lot of money to the hospital.

On another occasion McDonald's burger bar sent round some of their staff, dressed up in costumes. One of them, of course, was dressed up as Ronald McDonald. They did magic for the children, and held competitions. Then the person dressed as Ronald McDonald talked to every child individually and did some magic with each one. He could only talk to Rachel through the glass but he spent quite a long time chatting to her and was very impressed with her drawings, asking if he might have a photocopy for his shop. Rachel, of course, was eager to oblige. Then they gave presents to everyone, colouring books, crayons and felt-tips, as well as Get Well cards incorporating a token for a free burger and milk-shake. It made for a very enjoyable afternoon, and certainly cheered up the children.

So days passed, each one with a complete check-up from head to toe and blood tests. Occasionally she had a high temperature and when this happened it was panic stations. Because of her low blood count any infection could prove fatal if not dealt with immediately, so a raised temperature required samples of everything. Luckily she never did have an infection and towards the end she would say, 'Don't panic. I'm all right – you needn't bother with all this.' But the doctors would carry on just the same and when her results came back OK, Miss Muffett would say, 'See, I told you I was all right.' But she was very grateful that they were so quick to react, just in case.

On one occasion the doctors were a little worried that Rachel's chest might be infected but could detect nothing with their stethoscopes. They wanted to do a chest X-ray, but X-ray machines are covered in germs and cannot possibly be sprayed, so the doctors asked me if she could go to X-ray on the second floor. Sister Jane and I were not at all happy about this. Initially I said no, but then the doctors explained that if she did have an infection, by the time they could detect it with their stethoscopes it might be too late. Again I felt over a barrel: Do nothing and I could be putting her in danger; take her out of barrier and I could be putting her in danger. Hospitals are the worst place for germs.

I talked to Rachel about it and of course she wanted to go to X-ray. To get out of that room was exciting, it was like an outing for her. So I decided to take her. She was masked, gowned and gloved, and thought it was great fun. X-ray was alerted to clear the room so that we could go straight in. Rachel wanted to stroll up to the second floor, but she was bundled into a wheelchair pushed by the nurse, and I ran along beside her with the drip-stand. We whizzed up the corridors into the lifts waiting for us and dashed into X-ray. Rachel was laughing all the way. On reflection, we must have made quite a picture for other patients: a nurse running with a patient in a wheelchair in hysterics and covered from head to toe apart from two eyes; and a Mum chasing alongside with a drip-stand, also having hysterics. We had never before had such a quick X-ray and then it was another mad dash back to the ward.

When we arrived back I had to strip off Rachel's clothes and wash her all over, just as a precaution, and then she put on a complete outfit of clean clothes. Rachel thoroughly enjoyed her outing, but the nurse and I were shattered from the physical and mental strain of getting her there and back without contact with too many people. After the X-ray was seen by the doctors they announced that her chest was clear and everything was fine. That jaunt out of the ward had no bad effects on Rachel, I am pleased to say.

Days passed and one morning the doctor came down waving Rachel's blood count sheet, saying 'You can come out of barrier.' Rachel burst into tears and so did I.

At first she was only allowed out on to the ward without mixing with the other patients. The ward was designed with two bays, each holding about eight beds. At the time when Rachel was allowed out of barrier the ward was not very busy, so the nurses put all the other children in one bay while Rachel was allowed out for a stroll. I still had to keep up with the normal reverse barrier nursing procedures for her cubicle, but we were allowed to go in without masks and gowns. It was strange at first. On Rachel's first afternoon out of her cubicle she asked if she could make cakes in the kitchen for all the children for tea, so off I went to the local shops for some cake mixes and soon there were forty or so buns waiting for doctors, nurses and patients, Mums and Dads. She had iced some and decorated others with sweets. They disappeared faster than you could say cakes. Cathy, Rachel's consultant, said, 'Don't overdo things, Rachel. You will find that you get tired very easily.' But she might have been talking to the wall. Rachel had her freedom and was off. After her baking session she went back to her cubicle, a tired but very pleased little girl.

Gradually as time passed we were allowed to stop more and more of the precautionary chores. Then Sister Jane announced, 'If you want to, you can sleep on the ward tonight.' Within minutes Rachel had picked her spot next to her friend Claire and we transferred all her belongings on to the main ward. She was thrilled. It was heaven for her to be able to join in with other patients, to watch the television and video with others and to go into the playroom and play with new things, and to be able to play with someone else other than her Mum and Dad. It was nice to watch her nattering with her friend Claire who was about her age.

Another novelty for Rachel was that she could now have some new visitors. My Mum and Dad and sister and brother-in-law came to see her, but she only had eyes for her Grand-dad. They would laugh and tease each other all the time. Another visitor was her Uncle Rod; my brother-in-law. He had visited regularly while she had been in barrier as he worked in London once a week, but now it was nice to come 'for a hands-on visit and a kiss', he would say. He always bought a newsy card from Aunty Ann, who had written every other day to Rachel while she had been in barrier. Rachel used to call Rod 'Postman Pat', and looked forward to his visits to break up the routine of having just me, Pete and John.

Katy was now allowed to visit 'in the flesh'. She had had to stay out of the cubicle and had only been able to talk to her sister through the glass. It had been felt that Katy would be an added risk, being at school where there were so many germs. She had only been able to visit at weekends, and she didn't much like having to talk over the intercom. But now she could come and be close to Rachel, and was able to give her all the gossip about school and friends that Mums and Dads shouldn't hear. It was nice for me to have some real contact with Katy too, instead of over the telephone. I used to ring her every evening to give her an update on Rachel and find out what she had been doing at school and if she was being good for her Gran and Granddad. My Mum and Dad always said she had been no trouble to them. Considering the weird sort of life she was living – a Mum at the end of a telephone, a Dad who would come in so late she was asleep and go again before she woke up, and who left messages for her to wake up to, and living with grandparents in her own home – she coped really well and we had the best school report possible from her. Obviously, the way Katy coped with her sister being seriously ill was to immerse herself in her school work, trying to forget what was going on at home and hospital.

Both our children have always enjoyed school and they are both intelligent and bright. Rachel did school work that had been sent to her, even in the barrier cubicle for an hour mornings and afternoons. School work rather went to pot after she came out of barrier, and who could blame her after being cooped up for so long? She just wanted to join in with the other children and play games and watch the video, so I let her do just as she liked. I felt she had earned her freedom and school work could be forgotten for a while.

March came and Rachel's blood counts were slowly getting back to normal. Everything was looking good, except for the wretched platelets which did not multiply. For some reason they would not take off like the rest of her system and she had to be transfused regularly with them. They help the blood to clot and without any the smallest cut could cause serious bleeding. For me this was the most frustrating period of Rachel's treatment, because in every other way she was a picture of health, full of energy and raring to go home. After seeing her so restricted for so long I wanted her to enjoy as much pain-free time as she could, at home, doing what she wanted. Days passed and as the results came back with still no platelets she became depressed. Sometimes the platelets would creep up and with them our hopes, and then they would disappear again.

At one point the platelets were almost there, and Cathy said she could go home the next day if all was well. All Rachel heard was that she could go home. The next day the count had plummeted again. Rachel was heart-broken. Cathy felt so guilty at raising Rachel's hopes that she bought her a little gift to say she was sorry. It was very unsettling for all of us, but most of all for Rachel who was desperate to get home. Since she had come out of barrier I had been going home for the odd night here and there but poor Rachel had been in hospital for six weeks by this time, four or five of them in her cubicle completely isolated.

Rachel was transfused regularly with platelets to the level the doctors felt was safe for her, but by the next morning they had all disappeared again and we were back to square one (platelets live only for twenty-four hours). Sometimes after a transfusion I took her for a little walk outside the hospital, perhaps to the shops, or to feed the fish in the pond in the hospital grounds, but there was not much to do in the immediate vicinity and I wasn't allowed to take her too far away from the hospital. After a while, going out didn't hold much excitement for us.

As the days passed the platelets started to creep up again and this time they seemed to be holding. There was great excitement all round. Rachel's consultant had been to see us and told us that if the platelets did not come through soon, she would have to do a bone marrow test which involved sticking a needle in Rachel's back and drawing off some of the bone marrow. Neither of us liked the sound of this much, after all she had been down that road before and she didn't want to have to repeat it. However, a couple of days after being told this, Rachel's platelets started to stabilize. I think it must have been through sheer fright!

At last we could think about going home. Because Rachel's platelets would still be very low, and she would be prone to bruising very easily, we had been told that public transport was now out of the question. Although we had a car, I was the only driver, and although I had been driving for more than seventeen years I had never ventured into London. The very thought of it terrified me, but my father-in-law and brother-in-law, who have nerves of steel and are patience personified, offered to take it in turns to sit with me until I got used to the route and was confident I could do it with Rachel alone. This was soon achieved to my great satisfaction.

After I had got my confidence with the car, I was able to take Rachel further afield as her platelets slowly crept up. I kept the car at the hospital and in the afternoons we could go out if the doctors didn't want us for anything. One such afternoon we bundled into the car and took off to see Granny and Granddad Davies who lived at Beckenham. It was so nice for Rachel to have somewhere else to go and someone else to see. Granny and Granddad of course were delighted, so we sat in the garden and whiled away the afternoon, trying to forget the hospital and all that it entailed.

We were now nearing my birthday, 15 March, and we wanted to be at home for this, but the doctors would not permit it until Rachel's platelets had reached a certain level. On the night before my birthday, the ward sister allowed Peter and Katy to stay with me so that we were all together. When we woke up we went to find Rachel. As we walked on to the ward all the children began to sing 'Happy Birthday'. They had drawn me birthday cards secretly. I was overcome by the thoughtfulness and kindness the children were extending to me when they themselves were so poorly. I was given my presents and there was much excitement. Then Staff Nurse Kay told me I should go and make myself look nice and put on some make-up and ordered Rachel to have her bath. We couldn't understand what all the hurry was and were loathe to rush about when all we could do was sit around the hospital all day. But we did as we were told.

Rachel's daily blood test showed that the platelets were still stable, but too low for her Mum and Dad to take her out; she would be allowed out only with qualified nursing staff in attendance. As it was a Sunday there was fat chance of that, or so we thought. However, after a lot of to-ing and fro-ing who should appear but the ward sister and two staff nurses who were supposed to be off duty, and then the play worker who didn't work weekends, all dressed up in their Sunday best, telling us to hurry.

Rachel and I were baffled but Katy and Peter had little smirks on their faces. 'What's going on?' we said. 'We're off to feed the deer in the park,' Sister Jane announced. 'Oh, goody,' said Rachel and off we went. Sister Jane took us to her car and the others followed. After a drive around London we ended up in a back street. Sister Jane announced that we were going to get bread to feed the deer with, so we obediently followed her – only to find ourselves in the foyer of the Savoy Hotel! We had been brought here for breakfast as my birthday treat from Peter. It was a surprise for Rachel too, and we were overwhelmed by the kindness of the nurses who had given up their free time to enable Peter to take his family out for a treat. Rachel had her trained nurses with her in case of accident, and we had the most marvellous breakfast ever. The surroundings were exquisite and the food was delicious. Rachel especially appreciated it after hospital food for so long. A thoroughly good time was had by all, and after we had filled ourselves fit to burst these lovely ladies took us back to the hospital.

We didn't eat another thing all day. It was a lovely surprise and something I shall never forget. I think one of the best things was to see Rachel eating something and enjoying it. Her appetite had gone downhill of late. I thought it was just being in hospital and not being able to do much to work up an appetite; also, the diet in hospital left much to be desired, although I was allowed to cook meals and did so quite often. There didn't seem too much wrong with her appetite that day.

On reflection I wonder if she was just losing her battle against her disease. I asked the doctors so many times to check her out because her appetite had always been extremely good. They could not come up with any medical explanation and said it would right itself when she had settled down at home again. I accepted what they said, but it still used to worry me. Perhaps I was becoming over-anxious and over-protective, I don't know.

Another of our escapades while we were waiting for these wretched platelets to sort themselves out, was to decorate the parents' room. I offered to give the walls a coat of emulsion one evening as Sister Jane had been given a donation from a previous patient's family and she had decided it would be nice to clean it up a bit with a coat of paint and some new carpet tiles. So one evening, after Rachel had settled down for the night, I proceeded to paint the parents' room. I finished at 2 A.M. and went off to bed rather pleased with my efforts. It was a nice feeling to be able to do something for the nurses, after they had done so much for us.

Next morning Sister Jane came on to the ward. She was very pleased with what I had done, and promptly gave Rachel a black felt-tip marker, asking her if she would like to do one of her lovely drawings on the wall. Rachel was thrilled and went off to start her masterpiece. She drew hills and dales, trees and flowers that went the complete length of the room. She drew a pond with ducks on, and some little creatures of her own imagination called quirms. This took her most of the day. When she showed Sister Jane, she was asked if she would like to enlist some help from the other patients to paint what she had drawn. This she readily organized. They all decided what they wanted to paint and what colours they needed and off they went. During the evening of the next day it was beginning to look lovely and when Peter arrived to see us, Rachel asked him if he would get up on a chair and paint her sun shining in the sky.

Now my husband, bless him, is not a small man, and he was eager to get on with the job so he stood on a flimsy piece of wood across the arms of a chair. He was happily painting the sunshine when suddenly there was a crack, followed by hoots of laughter. I heard the story, when I returned from shopping nearby, to find my husband minus his shirt and shoes, with a very red-faced nurse. He had gone straight through the piece of wood, throwing the can of bright yellow paint all down his shirt, trousers and shoes. Rachel thought this was hilarious, and was full of giggles. The nurse was panic-stricken and ripped off Pete's shirt as the paint was the type that did not wash out. Another took his shoes and tried to get it off them. All their efforts could not save the shirt or shoes, and Pete wasn't prepared to let them try the trousers, so he had to go home in one of my shirts, which again caused great hilarity. This was a great talking point on the ward for the next couple of days.

Rachel and her friends completed the rest of the painting and the result was magnificent. This completed, she decided it would be nice to have a weeping willow on another wall with a picnic laid out beneath on a chequered cloth. The tree was finished, but the picnic underneath was not, when she was finally told, 'You can go home, Rachel.' As far as Rachel was concerned, that was that. The painting could wait.

On 18 March Rachel and I set off for home. Her Uncle Rod, Aunty Ann and cousin Sarah came to collect us. Rachel was still not allowed to mix with too many people at one time, and those she did mix with had to be in tip-top condition, so public transport was out of the question. Rachel was going home after spending sixty-two nights in the hospital. The excitement was overwhelming and she felt sick in the car on our homeward journey.

When she got home, she looked so happy. She went to see her rabbit Clover and her bedroom which Gran had got ready for her return, and she was in her element. She wanted nothing else. She was happy and content to be at home at last. It was heaven just to be all together again after so long.

CHAPTER EIGHT

WE HAD TO GO BACK to the hospital for regular blood checks to make sure all her levels were satisfactory and this we did a couple of times. During the days that followed Rachel and I would potter about at home and perhaps take a short drive in the afternoons and then pick Katy up from school. Sometimes Rachel's friends would come round after school, if they were well, and catch her up on all the gossip. At weekends we would go here and there, not too far afield because Rachel would tire easily. After being away from home for so long she was still revelling in being with her own things and, being a very contented child anyway, she would occupy herself for hours with all her different hobbies. She was always collecting something: keyrings, soaps, miniature ornaments – you name it, she collected it. She was also a keen musician and had an electric organ which she often played.

One afternoon Rachel and I took a ride to a local garden centre and she asked if she could buy herself a goldfish. As she had been so good in hospital I said she could, so she bought a goldfish bowl, some weed, stones and fish food. The lady in the garden centre said she should take all these things home, filling the bowl and letting the water stand for twenty-four hours before putting her goldfish in. This she duly did and when we returned at the weekend for the goldfish, she took a long time before she chose the one she wanted. On the way home in the car, clutching her goldfish in the plastic bag, she was wondering what to call him. After several obvious names for fish, such as Jaws, she decided on Flash, a naughty nickname she had for her Granddad. She would tease him for walking and driving slowly and say, 'Come on, Flash.' My Dad was amused by this. She adored him and used to tease him, as he did her, but in a loving way.

Now we were all together again at home, life began to settle down. Rachel and I went to Charing Cross Hospital two or three times a week, and each time she had a thorough check-up. All seemed to be going well and it was now nearing her birthday, 2 April. We arranged for her to have some of her friends visit for the evening, and some friends from the hospital came too. She had a birthday cake and played her favourite tapes and we all had a lovely evening. It was amazing to see Rachel disco-dancing with her friends when three months before she could at times hardly stand on her very swollen and painful leg. By the end of the evening she was exhausted, but she was so happy that she had had her birthday at home. She went off to bed very tired, but very content.

We had to go to the hospital the next day for a check-up, and when her blood test came back they said she would have to stay in for a blood transfusion. Rachel was not too happy. As she had just got used to being home again, Sister Jane assured her that we could go home the next day, which we did. It was Saturday 4 April, two days after Rachel's birthday. We arrived home about lunchtime and, after we had finished our lunch, Rachel settled down to look at her birthday presents. She had received quite a lot of money from various people; because she had had so many gifts sent to her in hospital, it was difficult for people to know what to buy her. After a short rest she asked if we could go into town to spend some of her money. She wanted an electronic keyboard and a new calculator for school, so we took off on a shopping spree. She found just the keyboard she wanted and the calculator too. Then she began to feel tired and we went home. At home she had a cup of tea and then played with her new keyboard, content to be at home with her family enjoying the aftermath of her birthday.

The next time we went for a check-up was 10 April. This time my sister Ann came with us for company. Rachel had her usual blood checks and while we were waiting for the results, I asked Sister Jane if she would mind having a look at Rachel's Hickman Line site, as it didn't look quite right to me. She said that it had started to slip out. Cathy the consultant decided it would be best if it were removed altogether as she didn't want it to fall out when we were at home.

The method used for Hickman Line insertion differs from hospital to hospital. In the Westminster when a line is inserted into a child it is done in such a way that it can be pulled out on the ward, with a local anaesthetic, but the Charing Cross has a different method. The line is held in with a inflatable collar under the skin and this means a mini-operation to remove it under a general anaesthetic. When Rachel learned of this she was petrified, and also very cross with me for drawing Sister's attention to it in the first place. Preparations were made for the removal of the line that same afternoon, but we were told that Rachel would have to stay in overnight because of the anaesthetic. My sister was allowed to stay with me and we settled down to coax and distract Rachel from what was to come. She had her pre-med after a second try – the first one was vomited up as soon as it went down, I think because she was so frightened. After a while she began to drift off to sleep, until she heard the trolley coming for her. I went with her as far as the lift to the theatre. The Charing Cross does not allow mothers into the ante-room, so I left her at the lift, and told her I would be waiting there when she came back.

I felt so guilty about mentioning the wretched line to the Sister. If I had not asked her to look at it she would never have known it had moved, but then I might have been putting Rachel at more risk had I not noticed something was wrong. After about half an hour Rachel was ready to come back to the ward. I was waiting at the lift expecting to hear the usual crying and screaming, but as the doors opened I saw my little girl beaming from ear to ear, saying, 'They do the operations in this hospital much better than the Westminster.' And that was that. After a while she wanted a drink and then turned over and went to sleep for the night. My sister and I went and had a coffee and cigarette and then decided to turn in for the night so we could get an early start for home the next day. Off we went to the playroom, mattresses in hand, back to the old routine.

Next day Rachel woke up and was eager to get going on the homeward journey. The doctors decided to take a precautionary blood test just to make sure her platelets were satisfactory, as she might have lost a few from bruising due to line removal. The blood test came back fine and so, without a moment to lose, we went to the car park and started for home. Without Rachel's line we could go swimming again and she was eager for the wound to heal so she could get back to doing all her favourite things. She had a couple of stitches this time so the healing would take a little longer, but she still felt free no longer having this thing dangling in front, and she had forgiven me for asking Sister

70

Jane to have a look at it. We dropped Aunty Ann at her house and then came home to a lovely dinner that Peter had cooked for us.

During the days that followed Rachel became increasingly pale and her appetite went haywire again. I had to bribe her to eat. She said she just didn't feel hungry. She also became very tired. I was worried about her so I rang the hospital and spoke to Sister Jane who said it would be a good idea for them to take a look at her. I was in the doghouse with Rachel again but I didn't want anything to go wrong now we were on the homeward stretch. After all she had been through it would be silly to let things slip now, so the next day we went for another check-up.

Rachel was quite worked up about going, because I think she felt that something was not quite right and she was afraid they might take her in again. She was right. They kept us in, but just for one night. After giving her a blood test they found her red cell count had gone down and she was in need of a blood transfusion. She cheered up when she found out what the trouble was and that she could go home the next day. Then we realized she had no Hickman Line, so this time it meant having a drip put in her arm, but as always she went through with it with hardly a complaint. After the last weeks she just wanted to be left alone to get her strength back, but because of the treatment she had been given her own system needed a boost from time to time.

The next morning we went home again. Rachel was much livelier, had a lovely little pink face and looked much better altogether, so much so that at the weekend we went to a funfair. I told Rachel that she was not going to be allowed to go on any of the fast rides but she was quite content to spend her money and time on the side-shows. She decided she would try and win Katy a present, so she threw darts to win a goldfish. Flash needed a friend, she thought, and it would be nice for Katy to have a fish too. It was 50p a go and each time she nearly made it but not quite. After the third try she decided to enlist her Dad's help. 'This one must really be made of gold,' said Pete, as £2 seemed over the going rate for a goldfish, but Rachel was pleased as punch, and immediately gave the fish to Katy. Now the name-choosing began again. Katy wanted Nick, Rachel wanted Sparky, and they started to argue just like always. It was lovely to hear them being like normal sisters again. As soon as Rachel began to tire we came home, but we had enjoyed such a happy time.

Rachel seemed on the up and up again and we continued with our visits to London for check-ups. I had had a part-time secretarial job four mornings a week before Rachel had become ill and when I explained to my boss what was happening, he told me to go and get Rachel well, and not to worry about my job. I could give no clues as to how long I would be away, so we left it at that, if they could hold my job for me they would, but if too much time went by they might have to get a replacement. As time passed, Rachel seemed to be on the mend so I went back to my job for a couple of weeks and Rachel managed a week back at school. She coped very well, although it tired her out. She wanted to return to Guides and Red Cross, but by the end of a school day she was whacked and spent the evenings relaxing and watching television. Our next-door neighbours were two retired ladies who loved Rachel to go in and have a natter with them. They also took her out a couple of times to local Garden Centres. Rachel loved to visit them and show them all the different things she had made, looking at photographs and the like, so some mornings I went off to work knowing Rachel was quite happy and safe with these two kind ladies.

Rachel enjoyed her week at school and then, much to her disappointment, it was time to break up for Easter. 'Typical,' she said, 'just when I'm ready to go back to school it's the holidays.' Still, she had got back into the swing of school and could enjoy the holidays with her sister and do as she liked. We were hopeful that she would be able to go back to normal schooling after the Easter break. She had certainly proved she could cope and by then she would be that bit more rested and stronger. She came home proudly saying that she hadn't missed much and would be able to go back without any worries about being behind the others. She had a very positive attitude and school work presented no worries; it was something she really enjoyed and if Rachel enjoyed something she did her best. She told us about the homework for the holidays, 'I'll soon have this done,' was her attitude – and she did.

We had to make another trip to Charing Cross Hospital on 15 April. Pete took a day off to take her so that I could go to work and then prepare dinner. When I arrived home at about 1 P.M. I rang the ward to see how long they would be. I spoke to Sister Jane who said Pete had just taken Rachel to ultrasound and that things weren't looking too good. I was speechless. She explained that they had immediately noticed that Rachel was looking jaundiced. I suppose we had got so used to her pale face that we hadn't noticed. She had not complained of feeling unwell and seemed to have plenty of energy. When Pete had walked her to the station that morning she had complained of feeling breathless, but he assumed that was because she was nervous about going back to the hospital.

When he arrived on the ward with her, the usual tests

were done and the doctors decided to do an ultrasound scan as well. They were concerned that her colour could indicate that all was not well with her liver. Sister Jane suggested I should pack a bag and come immediately.

CHAPTER NINE

AFTER I PUT THE PHONE DOWN I rushed around the house packing a bag for Rachel and myself. Why had things got to go wrong now? Why couldn't she get better and be left in peace to enjoy the pain-free time the doctors had so far been able to give her? I remember saying, 'Bless her heart, please don't let there be anything serious wrong. Please God, give her a break.' She had been through enough. We had all been praying constantly for her recovery and I remember spluttering through my tears, 'Dear God, if you are not going to let her get well, then take her. Please, please don't make her suffer any more. She's done everything to try and get better, so, please, she's suffered enough.'

I pulled myself together, put on some more war-paint and set off to London to find my family. When I arrived the good news was that Rachel's liver was OK, it did not seem to have been damaged in any way by the treatment, and they could not detect any cancer which the doctors had been afraid might have been the reason for her jaundiced colour. The bad news was that we had to stay in because the doctors were far from happy with the laboratory results. They could not understand why Rachel was showing signs of jaundice. Of the four possible causes, two had already been dismissed by the ultrasound, there was no sign of mestastasis (spreading of the cancer) and the liver was not damaged due to BCNU toxicity. (It was possible that any of Rachel's organs could have been damaged during the treatment – but it was a risk we had to take.)

The doctors were confused and thought she might have hepatitis from an infected transfusion, although they assured us it was most unlikely as all bloods were screened. It could be incompatibility with the transfusion – they just didn't know. Because of the hepatitis risk to other patients, we were put straight back into barrier. We were back to square one, and both very upset as we didn't know how long it was going to take them to find out what was causing the liver malfunction. She had some more tests done and we just had to wait for the results. Pete took Katy home and Rach and I stayed in barrier and went back to our old routine of playing games and watching television.

Then some more good news: it was not hepatitis, so the barrier was not necessary. Gradually Rachel's colour began to return to normal, but she was still very pale. The yellowy look was going, although she still was breathless after exertion. The doctors felt this was likely to be due to anxiety as they could find no medical reason for it. To all intents and purposes everything was working properly. So, reassured that her liver was functioning correctly after all and dismissing the four suspected reasons for the liver malfunction, we were told we could go home again. I had gone home the night before and driven up the next morning to collect Rachel as she felt she could not cope with the trains. She seemed very tired but much happier once she was home again. She was still getting breathless when she did anything much, but we felt confident that the doctors had looked her over and felt that it might indeed just be anxiety. All the feelings she had experienced over the last eight weeks had to come out somewhere. She had been so good and accepted everything that had been done to her with no trouble at all. I comforted myself with the thought that the doctors wouldn't send us home if they had any doubts at all. I trusted them completely; they had always been truthful before and I didn't feel they would keep things from me now. After all they had done for Rachel, they wouldn't take chances with her now.

We pottered about at home and did whatever Rachel felt she could cope with. Her appetite still left much to be desired and this worried me because she had been losing weight steadily throughout the eight weeks. She had always been plump and could afford to lose some of the weight, but I didn't want her to lose much more. She developed a cough, a silly dry cough that seemed to niggle. She felt that if she could have a proper cough it would go away, but she seemed unable to do that. After a couple of days she seemed to have breathless attacks, spasms, a bit like asthma. This was the one thing I could not cope with and I would panic too, trying to breathe for her, which made her worse. Peter saved the day because he had suffered with asthma and knew what it was like, so he could calm Rachel very easily. He would sit quietly and talk to her and soon her breathing would return to normal.

We rang Charing Cross and they said they would like to see her, so up we went again on 21 April, bag in hand, as they told us that it was likely we would have to stay. Rachel had all the tests on her chest again and the doctors prepared for an arterial blood test. None of them liked doing this test because it was painful, but blood taken from an artery enables them to measure the level of blood gases. It was hoped it would give them a medical reason for Rachel's breathlessness. Her favourite doctor Naz was really upset that he had to do this to Rachel. He told her he was going to hurt her, but that he would try and get it done as quickly as possible.

Rachel co-operated. She trusted Naz implicitly and knew he would do the best for her, but, hard as he tried, he could not get the needle in the right place. Finally, very upset himself, he said, 'Rachel, I can't do this to you any more. I will have to get someone else to help me.' Another doctor, Mitch, came in and explained he would do his best not to hurt her any more than necessary. He started to insert the needle and Rachel screamed and held on to me tightly. I did my best to comfort her. Eventually it was done, the doctors got the blood they required and Rachel was left alone to recover. She soon got over the upset and was playing a board game with me, Pete and Kate, saying, 'They are not doing that to me again, so there.'

With the tests completed the doctors were still puzzled by Rachel's bouts of breathlessness and told us they had two ideas: BCNU toxicity or anxiety. Their opinion was that her lungs might have been slightly damaged by the BCNU, and that Rachel's anxiety was making things worse. After all the tests were completed they felt that there was nothing untoward going on, they decided we could go home again. They said, 'If you are worried at all about her or she worsens in any way, just ring and we'll see her.' We made a provisional appointment to return on 5 May for some lung function tests to ascertain whether Rachel's lungs would be up to another course of treatment at a later date, should she require it.

On the way home Rachel said she wanted to go to Gran and Granddad Davies at Beckenham to say hello to them and the dog and to reassure them that she was all right. When we finally arrived home Rachel was still breathless after any exertion, but she wanted to ring her Gran and Granddad Denton and invite them for a cup of tea. Mum and Dad came straight away and were pleased to see that she was looking all right, although they too were worried about how breathless she got. But, as Mum said, 'If the doctors aren't worried, then there can't be much wrong with her.' I comforted myself with the thought that perhaps we were all suffering from anxiety.

Rachel spent the afternoon nattering with her grandparents and after they had gone home she watched television, saying she was feeling much better. Peter and I were naturally worried and watched her very carefully. As long as she was sitting still she was fine, but when she went upstairs or walked too fast she seemed to get out of breath. She still got those little spasms of breathlessness, too, but Pete would be at her side talking to her calmly and she would soon recover.

The next day, Saturday 25 April, Rachel wanted her Aunty Ann and Uncle Rod to come and see her. They brought the dogs, Crackers and Ritzy. Rachel loved animals and she spent a pleasant evening with them. But climbing the stairs at bedtime brought the panic back and Pete had to talk her through it as usual. The doctors had prescribed steroid tablets to ease her breathing problems, and they seemed to have helped, but they have side-effects and can upset the stomach. There was also medicine to counteract the side-effects. Rachel didn't like the medicine much and I wasn't too happy about the steroids, but I was assured it was a low dose and could be helpful, so I continued with her medication when we got home as instructed. We settled Rachel down for the night and she had a good night's rest.

In the morning, Sunday 26 April, I was woken by Rachel coughing and crying. I jumped out of bed and found her in the bathroom, very breathless and upset. Pete was by my side in a flash and started to calm her, as only he could do. We got her back to bed and she started to explain that she had woken up and wanted to go to the loo. She had become frightened and breathless and that woke us up. We told her she should have called us before she got up so we could have been with her, but in her usual way she had said, 'I didn't want to wake you up, because you're both so tired and need your rest.' (She was always so thoughtful of others.)

Once she had settled in bed, Peter and I tried to explain what the doctors had told us about her lungs. It was hard enough for us to understand; could she understand that she might be making things worse by being over-anxious? She said she thought she understood and that she would try not to get in a panic.

Over the previous few days we had tried to get her to do things because the doctors had told us to keep her active, but she had reached the point where she was frightened to move for fear of losing her breath. I wanted to do everything for her so she wouldn't get frightened, but at the same time I didn't want her to give up – not after all she had been through. So we tried to be firm and to encourage her as much as we could. I felt so cruel.

After a cup of tea in bed and a small breakfast she said she would like to have a bath, but if she did she knew she would get out of breath. With a stern voice, but a wobbly tummy, I told her to think positive. If she wanted a bath, then she should have one – 'Dad and I are here at hand if you want us.' After much thought she decided to take her bath and was pleasantly surprised that it wasn't that bad. I helped her dry herself and dress, then she felt exhausted so I left her on her bed reading to recuperate. After a while she called, saying she wanted to come down to the garden and finish her homework as she was going to school the next day. Pete and I looked at each other in amazement, hoping our little chat with her had sunk in.

Pete went upstairs to walk her down to the garden, talking

to her all the time about everything under the sun except breathing. Halfway down, she started to panic and we told her to calm down and think positive. Easy for us to say but much harder for Rachel to do, and she did try very hard to be brave.

She settled in the garden quite happily doing her home-work and I asked her what she wanted for lunch. She said chicken risotto. I put hers on a tray and we sat in the conservatory to have lunch, but after a couple of mouthfuls she said she was full. I snapped, 'If you don't eat you'll lose your strength,' and I went on, 'If you lose your strength, you'll give up your fight.' I told her to pull herself together and push herself. I told her we were all trying to do our best for her but she must help herself. 'We can't fight for you on our own, you must keep on at your end.' On and on I went. I have since felt so guilty about that outburst. Poor little love, how dare I criticize such a brave soldier? She had been to hell and back, and now I was shouting at her. I would have folded at the first fence, but not Rachel. She had given her all.

I calmed down and knelt by her chair and said I was sorry. I asked her to forgive me. I asked her if she understood that outburst. She looked at me and smiled, 'Of course I do, Mum,' she said. 'You're trying to make me fight with you to get rid of my anxiety, which will help me calm down inside and that will help my breathing.' What a child. She said, 'How can I get cross with people who love and and try to help me?' I felt ashamed. I told her it was because I loved her so much that I had gone on at her and she said she understood. We kissed and made up. She went back to her homework and I went back to the dishes. At this time I was so afraid that we were going to lose the battle because

Rachel, who had been the strongest of us all, seemed in danger of giving in now we were over the worst.

Chores done, we were all sitting in the garden when Rachel asked if her friend Diane could come round to play. Peter and I thought she might relax nattering with her chum, and within half an hour Diane had arrived. Rachel wanted to go to her bedroom to listen to her stereo and chat, but on climbing the stairs she had another attack which frightened Diane. Pete was at her side in no time and he helped her up the stairs. They played quite happily all afternoon once settled in her room. I took some drinks up later, and they had ice-lollies.

At about 6 o'clock I went up to see what they were doing. Rachel looked very tired and was breathing more heavily, even though she was lying down. I told Pete and we rang the hospital without telling Rachel. Dr Louise was on duty and I told her all about Rachel's breathing which seemed to be getting heavier. She said she had read all Rachel's notes and that she didn't think there was need for worry, but, as always, if I wanted to take her up she would be willing to see her. I also asked if I could stop giving her the steroids as she had been complaining of tummy ache and feeling sick. She said that was all right and that if we were worried we should ring again. If not, she would see us the next day for a check-up.

I took Diane home and I suggested to Rachel that she have an early night and get ready for bed. 'Oh, Mum, I'm so tired I can't be bothered to get undressed. I'll just have a little sleep then come down and watch telly,' she said. I settled her down and kept a watchful eye on her. After a while she went to sleep and her breathing, although still rapid, seemed less laboured. During the evening Pete or I popped up to check and she seemed quite peaceful. After an hour or more we felt she had gone off for the night. Peter came up to help me undress her without waking her, but unfortunately she did wake. We put her in her night clothes and settled her down again.

We had upset her breathing again, and then she needed to go to the loo, which made her breathing even worse. Peter started to calm her, but this time it didn't work. I rang the Charing Cross Hospital again and explained that Rachel's breathing seemed to be worsening. Dr Louise listened carefully and agreed that I should call our GP. She said the GP could ring her for a medical update. I rang our GP and while we were waiting I explained to Rachel what I had done. She said she would like to see a doctor as she was frightened. Even Peter, always so calm and collected, was like a jelly inside.

Dr Anderson, who knew all about Rachel although he was not our GP, arrived and found a very distressed little girl, who immediately shouted at him do something. He gave her a full examination while I gave him a run-down of events, treatment and blood counts. He sat and talked to Rachel and explained that her lungs were working and she had no infection or fluid build-up. He could hear the air getting into her lungs and told her that she must try to relax by mentally putting parts of her body to sleep, starting with her toes. She listened intently to him and tried to follow what he was saying. She began to calm slightly. Dr Anderson told Pete to carry on with her while he went to ring Charing Cross. Downstairs I asked him what was wrong with Rachel. He said he didn't think there was too much to worry about, but that she was obviously distressed and he would speak to Charing Cross for a complete medical update. I was about to get the number for him when Pete called and asked him to come.

Meanwhile poor Katy was in her bedroom, hearing all but understanding nothing. I had completely forgotten about her. Peter and I went into her and tried to explain what the doctor was doing to Rachel. We were all in a state of utter confusion. I left Pete with Kate and went back to Rachel, and I think I knew then that my baby had died. Finally he said that he could do nothing more. Those dreaded words.

CHAPTER TEN

I WENT BACK to Peter and Katy and told them. Katy exploded in anger, and Pete and I were numb.

No one expected Rachel to die. She fought so hard to live. She was such a loving thoughtful child, and she was gone. She was now at peace, and no one could harm her any more.

Dr Anderson later told me that Rachel's death was inevitable (purely from the fact that she had secondaries in her spine), but not predictable. He could not explain why it happened. He certainly did not expect it to happen when he saw her earlier. We had been told to look on the treatment as buying time for her, but we had always maintained a positive approach and we were going for a cure in our own minds. When you are fighting with someone to overcome a cancer, you always think positive, just as Rachel certainly did – her attitude to her illness put us all to shame at times. But when the fights ends and you are faced with the awful truth, it hits you like a sledge-hammer. We all thought we were going to be the lucky ones and win.

I had promised Rachel I was going to write a book about her bravery and tell everyone how she fought her disease and won. And now I can't say we beat it, but Rachel certainly tried her darndest, and so I have written this book in Rachel's memory. I don't like the ending, she deserved to win. I want everyone to know how proud of her I am, and how privileged I feel to have been her mum. Mums are supposed to teach their children about life, but my little girl taught me. I love and miss her so much, but her memory lives on in the pages you have just read.

To anyone who has just been told they or their child has cancer, I would say, take comfort from Rachel and don't give up. During her illness we had good times, and now they are treasured memories for me, Peter and Katy. One day there will be a cure for cancer. I just wish Rachel could have been here for it.

CHAPTER ELEVEN

AFTER RACHEL'S DEATH, our world seemed to stop. People were coming and going to our house; doctors, funeral directors, churchmen, everyone came and went. I really don't remember much. The phone did not stop ringing, the postman pushed hundreds of sympathy cards and letters through the door, so much so that I dreaded the sight of him.

I wanted to die and be with Rachel. We were all offered tranquillizers, but we all refused; there was no pill to put us right. We functioned during the days that followed like robots. We arranged Rachel's funeral, and on the day were greeted by a sea of faces. To this day I could not tell you who was there and who was not. All I can remember is that I felt so empty, and hearing the Bob Marley song 'Two Little Birds' playing – a song I used to sing to Rachel, telling her it was her tune because of the words: don't worry about a thing 'cause every little thing's gonna be all right. Well it wasn't all right.

We found it very hard to cope. We hadn't realized the extent to which hospitals, appointments and check-ups had become our way of life. Now it had all stopped. We were three instead of four, everything we did seemed wrong. Even having a meal caused distress, seeing Rachel's empty place at the table. None of us could cope with sitting at the dining table, so we ate our meals on trays in front of the television, something I would never let the girls do because we always used mealtimes as a social event to talk about our days with each other. Now mealtimes just hurt.

Katy was distraught. She had lost her chum. She had no one to play with or fight with. They had been very close and she found it very hard to be on her own. She begged Pete and I to have a baby. 'Please, I want you to have a baby,' she would say. We tried to explain to her it wasn't a baby she wanted, it was Rachel. Slowly she came to realize that no one could replace Rachel and accepted that she may even have resented another child in the home being where Rachel should have been. We explained that we knew how she felt, and that she would have to be patient, and slowly she would adjust to these feelings. We would have to work through our feelings together and there was a tough time ahead, but we would pull through.

We had good days and bad days, but we had each other and we were lucky; we never all seemed to be down at the same time. The strong one could help the weak one, and as time passed we coped better. Katy went back to school, where she had a tough time. All their mutual friends took it on themselves to look after Katy at school, and when she came home some days she would howl for a while, just to let out all the emotions of the day. She was touched by her friends' kindness, but she kept a stiff-upper-lip all day at school, and then came home to have a good cry. She coped very well, and today she is a very capable young lady, and I'm very proud of her. She had a very strange childhood, coping with things far beyond her years, but she is now a well-adjusted and clever adult. She often says she feels Rachel's close to her and watching out for her, and I'm sure she's right.

For myself, I was terrified of having time alone with

nothing to do. I couldn't stop working, I couldn't allow myself time to sit and think – I felt I would go under if I did that – so I returned to work, ran my home and immersed myself in voluntary work, hardly allowing myself time to breathe. I can't remember how long this went on, but I know family and friends were becoming concerned for me and I was told frequently that I must slow down, I was heading for a breakdown. Yet I knew what I was doing, and told them I would slow down when I felt I could cope with it and not before. I can remember people crossing the street when they saw me coming, rather than having to talk to me. That used to hurt me so much as I needed to talk about Rachel, but others couldn't cope. I think they were afraid I would crumple on them, but they needn't have worried. I would go back home and, like Katy, howl and throw things around for a while and then compose myself again.

My husband Peter, in his normal manner, appeared most of the time to be in control of his emotions and was very strong and supportive. Inside I know it was different. He relived Rachel's final moments many times, seeing her smile, feeling his hand squeezed and then it stopping. A very large part of his life stopped at that time; he had taken my daughters as his own and now one had gone. An everyday event would reduce him to tears, but he would quickly cover up to protect me and Kate. One of the hardest things for him to cope with was when 'friends' would say, 'You'll get over it'. He didn't want to, because he felt that implied you had forgotten and he didn't want to forget. After a time you do lose sight of the bad bits and remember with great happiness the good bits. Peter returned to work and, like Katy and me, would release his pent-up feelings when he got home. Many an evening was spent with the three of us having a good cry, a laugh and sometimes a fight with each other, but at least we did it together, sorting each other out. Pete also joined the Red Cross, as he had promised Rachel he would join with her and Kate when she was better. He went on to become a Youth Leader of Rachel and Katy's group and is still involved with the movement. He has handed over the running of the youth group to Katy and her young man.

We used to, and still do sometimes, pick out a child that looks like Rachel. I think sometimes we are looking for her, but we take comfort in the fact that so many of the good things about Rachel are evident in others.

We found Christmas and birthdays, or any family celebration, very hard to cope with; there was always an empty space. We had to keep things as normal as possible for Katy who still had a lot of growing up to do, and we couldn't take that away from her. Christmas now for me is a time to get through, but we still continue to have our family get-togethers, and feel Rachel with us in spirit, along with her granddad Denton who died not long after Rachel. We often say, 'I expect they're still teasing and joking with each other, wherever they are.'

I can now sit quietly and relax and have time to think, recalling all the lovely things we did as a foursome and it brings Rachel back to me for a short while. I can cope. At least we still have our memories; they can never be taken away.

It's now six years since we lost our beloved Rachel. Life is easier to cope with, and Rachel will always be with us. You never get over losing someone you love, but you do learn to live alongside that loss. Life will never be the same for us, but we have coped, just like Rachel did.

USEFUL ADDRESSES

ACT Association for Children with Life-threatening Conditions and their Families
Institute of Child Health
Royal Hospital for Sick Children
St Michael's Hill
Bristol BS2 8BJ
Tel: 0272 221556

Provides an information resource on all services throughout the UK for children and young people with life-threatening conditions.

Cancer and Leukaemia in Childhood Trust
12/13 King Square
Bristol BS2 8JH
Tel: 01179 248844

Aims to help young people under 21 years who have any form of cancer or leukaemia and their families.

Cancer Relief Macmillan Fund
Anchor House
15/19 Britten Street
London SW3 3TZ
Tel: 0171 351 7811

Aims to help people cope with the effects of cancer. Establishes Macmillan cancer care nurses and Macmillan doctors: builds cancer day centres and gives grants to patients and families in financial difficulties.

Childhood Cancer and Leukaemia Link (CALL)
36 Knowles Avenue
Crowthorne
Berks RG11 6DU
Tel: 0344 750319

Support for parents of children who have cancer or leukaemia. Also will link up children with other children if they wish.

Compassionate Friends
53 North Street
Bristol
Avon BS3 1EN
Tel: 0272 539639

Offers friendship and support to grieving parents who have lost a child at any age.

CRUSE – Bereavement Care
Cruse House
126 Sheen Road
Richmond
Surrey TW9 1UR
Tel: 0181 940 4818

Offers help to all bereaved people through its 194 local branches by providing both individual and group counselling, opportunities for social contact and practical advice.

Health Information in the Weald
Sevenoaks Hospital
Hospital Road
Sevenoaks
Kent TN13 3PG
Tel: 0732 455155

An information service for people
with serious illness and those who
care for them.

Malcolm Sargent Cancer Fund
for Children
14 Abingdon Road
London W8 6AF
Tel: 0171 937 4548

Provides financial and other help for
families who have a young person
(under 21 years) suffering from any
form of cancer.

Society of Parents of Children
with Cancer
427 Reddings Lane
Hall Green
Birmingham B11 3DE
Tel: 021 777 9468

Support for families with children
with cancer through medical talks,
support meetings, newsletters, trips,
holidays, parent contact.

MAKE-A-WISH FOUNDATION® UK

The purpose of the Make-A-Wish Foundation is very simple – to grant the special wishes of children who suffer from life-threatening illnesses. We endeavour to provide the Wish Child and his/her family with memories to treasure which are filled with love, joy, and laughter – a time of just plain good fun! A time that is in total contrast to a life of hospitals, doctors and treatment. We believe doctors provide the treatment and Make-A-Wish provides the magic, in the hope that sometimes they might combine to produce a miracle!

It all began in Phoenix, Arizona in 1980 with a seven-year-old boy, suffering from leukaemia, who wanted to be a policeman. His local police force granted his wish by giving him his own badge, custom-made uniform and helmet and even his own miniature motorbike. The picture of happiness, he rode up and down the pavement and even handed out parking tickets to passers by. From that one small child's delight the Make-A-Wish Foundation was born.

Make-A-Wish Foundation is now the largest wishgranting organisation in the world, operating in the UK, Australia, Belgium, Canada, Chile, Holland, Ireland, Japan, New Zealand, Taiwan and the United States of America.

Make-A-Wish Foundation UK started in 1986 when our founder learnt of the work of the Foundation during a visit to the USA and was motivated to start up a UK organisation. It is now a national organisation directed by a volunteer Board of Trustees with its head office in Camberley, Surrey and eleven area offices. It has granted the wishes of hundreds of special children since it began and is now granting around 150 wishes per year.

Who can be a Wish Child? Any child, aged three to eighteen, suffering from a life-threatening illness can be referred to Make-A-Wish. We learn about a child from family, friends, teachers, medical personnel or clergy; in fact anyone can contact Make-A-Wish.

Make-A-Wish Foundation is unique in that we understand that the whole family feels the pain of a sick child. Furthermore, we understand that the happiness of the child's wish is increased when it is shared with parents, brothers and sisters. Therefore, we ensure that the family take part in the child's wish, with all expenses being met for the Wish Child, its parents and siblings up to age eighteen. By doing so, we hope to guarantee happy and precious memories for all.

Funding and support comes from all sorts of giving – Adopt-A-Wish, gifts in kind, corporate sponsors, covenants, payroll giving, group donation and the generous donation of time from our volunteers and associates. We want to build a wishgranting fund so that in future no child's special wish has to go ungranted through lack of finance.

Thank you for taking time to learn about the Make-A-Wish Foundation and our special children.

We welcome your support, as each one of us can influence the future success of this Foundation by talking about it to others so that they too can help to Make-A-Wish come true today, for a child who may have few tomorrows.

For further information contact:
Make-A-Wish Foundation UK
Suite B, Rossmore House
26-42 Park Street
Camberley, Surrey GU15 3PL
Tel: 0276 24127 Fax: 0276 683727